DATE DUE

Demco, Inc. 38-293

Headache in Children and Adolescents

Paul Winner, DO, FAAN, FAAP

Director, Palm Beach Headache Center
Co-Director, Premiere Research Institute
West Palm Beach, Florida
Clinical Associate Professor of Neurology
Nova Southeastern University
Fort Lauderdale, Florida

A. David Rothner, MD, FAAN, FAAP

Director Emeritus
Section of Child Neurology
Director, Pediatric/Adolescent Headache Program
Cleveland Clinic Foundation
Cleveland, Ohio

2001
B C DECKER INC
Hamilton • London

B C Decker Inc
20 Hughson Street South
P.O. Box 620, L.C.D. 1
Hamilton, Ontario L8N 3K7
Tel: 905-522-7017; 1-800-568-7281
Fax: 905-522-7839
E-mail: info@bcdecker.com
Website: www.bcdecker.com

WL
342
W 776h
2001

01 02 03 04 /UTP/ 9 8 7 6 5 4 3 2

ISBN 1–55009–125–5
Printed in Canada

Sales and Distribution

United States
B C Decker Inc
P.O. Box 785
Lewiston, NY 14092-0785
Tel: 905-522-7017; 1-800-568-7281
Fax: 905-522-7839
E-mail: info@bcdecker.com
Website: www.bcdecker.com

Canada
B C Decker Inc
20 Hughson Street South
P.O. Box 620, L.C.D. 1
Hamilton, Ontario L8N 3K7
Tel: 905-522-7017; 1-800-568-7281
Fax: 905-522-7839
E-mail: info@bcdecker.com
Website: www.bcdecker.com

Foreign Rights
John Scott & Company
International Publishers' Agency
P.O. Box 878
Kimberton, PA 19442
Tel: 610-827-1640
Fax: 610-827-1671

Japan
Igaku-Shoin Ltd.
Foreign Publications Department
3-24-17 Hongo
Bunkyo-ku,Tokyo, Japan 113-8719
Tel: 3 3817 5680; Fax: 3 3815 6776
E-mail: fd@igaku.shoin.co.jp

**U.K., Europe, Scandinavia,
Middle East**
Harcourt Publishers Limited
Customer Service Department
Foots Cray High Street
Sidcup, Kent
DA14 5HP, UK
Tel: 44 (0) 208 308 5760
Fax: 44 (0) 181 308 5702
E-mail: cservice@harcourt_brace.com

**Singapore, Malaysia, Thailand, Philippines,
Indonesia, Vietnam, Pacific Rim, Korea**
Harcourt Asia Pte Limited
583 Orchard Road
#09/01, Forum
Singapore 238884
Tel: 65-737-3593
Fax: 65-753-2145

Australia, New Zealand
Harcourt Australia Pty. Limited
Customer Service Department
STM Division
Locked Bag 16
St. Peters, New South Wales, 2044
Australia
Tel: (02) 9517-8999; Fax: (02) 9517-2249
E-mail: stmp@harcourt.com.au
Website: www.harcourt.com.au

Contributors

JACK GLADSTEIN, MD
Associate Dean for Student Affairs
Associate Professor of Pediatrics
Director, Pediatric Headache Clinic
University of Maryland, School of
    Medicine
Baltimore, Maryland

PETER J. GOADSBY, MD, DSc, FRACP,
    FRCP
Professor
Institute of Neurology
The National Hospital for Neurology
    and Neurosurgery
London, United Kingdom

ANDREW HERSHEY, MD, PhD
Assistant Professor of Pediatrics and
    Neurology
University of Cincinnati
Director, Headache Center
Cincinnati's Children's Hospital
    Medical Center
Cincinnati, Ohio

ALVIN E. LAKE III, PhD
Division Director of Behavioral
    Medicine
Associate Program Director of
    Head-Pain Treatment Unit
Michigan Head-Pain and
    Neurological Institute
Ann Arbor, Michigan

DONALD W. LEWIS, MD
Associate Professor of Pediatrics
    and Neurology
Eastern Virginia Medical School
Children's Hospital of the King's
    Daughters
Norfolk, Virginia

STEVEN L. LINDER, MD
Dallas Pediatric Neurology Associates
Assistant Clinical Professor
University of Texas Health Science
    Center of Dallas
Dallas, Texas

RICHARD LIPTON, MD
Professor of Neurology,
    Epidemiology, and Social
    Medicine
Albert Einstein College of Medicine
Montefiore Medical Center
Innovative Medical Research
Stamford, Connecticut

JOSEPH MAYTAL, MD
Professor of Clinical Neurology
    and Pediatrics
Chief, Pediatric Neurology
Schneider Children's Hospital
Albert Einstein College of Medicine
North Shore-Long Island Jewish
    Health System
New Hyde Park, New York

A. David Rothner, MD, FAAN,
   FAAP
Director Emeritus
Section of Child Neurology
Director, Pediatric/Adolescent
   Headache Program
Cleveland Clinic Foundation
Cleveland, Ohio

Stephen D. Silberstein, MD
Professor of Neurology
Thomas Jefferson University
Director, Jefferson Headache Center
Thomas Jefferson University Hospital
Philadelphia, Pennsylvania

Warren W. Wasiewski, MD
Director
Mayday Pediatric Headache Center
Lancaster, Pennsylvania

Paul Winner, DO, FAAN, FAAP
Director, Palm Beach Headache
   Center
Co-Director, Premiere Research
   Institute
West Palm Beach, Florida
Clinical Associate Professor of
   Neurology
Nova Southeastern University
Fort Lauderdale, Florida

Contents

Foreword   vii

Preface   ix

Introduction   xi

1   Epidemiology and Classification of Headache   1
Richard B. Lipton, Joseph Maytal, Paul Winner

2   Evaluation of Headache   20
A. David Rothner

3   Secondary Headaches   33
A. David Rothner, Andrew Hershey

4   Migraine Pathophysiology   47
Peter J. Goadsby

5   Migraine, Migraine Variants, and
Other Primary Headache Syndromes   60
Donald W. Lewis, Paul Winner

6   Pharmacologic Treatment of Headache   87
Paul Winner, Steven L. Linder, Warren W. Wasiewski

7   Chronic Daily Headache   116
Jack Gladstein, Paul Winner

8   Psychologic and Nonpharmacologic Treatment of Headache   126
Donald W. Lewis, Alvin E. Lake III

9   Post-traumatic Headache   142
Paul Winner, Stephen D. Silberstein

10   Miscellaneous Headache Syndromes   153
A. David Rothner

11   Headache in the Pediatric Emergency Department   163
Donald W. Lewis

Index   182

Foreword

Headache is common in children; however, until recently, there has been very little attention to this problem. Just as headache in women was once regarded as a manifestation of neurosis, this symptom in children was often assumed to be a ruse for avoiding school or chores. During the last two decades of the twentieth century, there have been major advances in understanding the mechanism and treatment of migraine, as well as other primary headaches.

Doctors Winner and Rothner are renown pediatric neurologists with special expertise in the field of headache. They have been major advocates for children with this condition. The information related in their book is clear and well organized. The authors draw not only on scientific developments, but also on their own extensive experience. This book will be a great help to pediatricians and all care givers who deal with headaches in children.

Seymour Solomon, MD
Director, Headache Unit
Albert Einstein College of Medicine/
Montefiore Medical Center

Preface

Children and adolescents experience significant pain and disability from headache. However, in most instances their pain and disability can be diagnosed swiftly and efficiently and relieved effectively.

This comprehensive, clinically oriented text, addressing the diagnostic and management aspects of headache in children and adolescents, intends to assist the practicing physician and health professional who face these issues regularly. The text offers practical solutions in an easy-to-understand format with clinical cases designed to punctuate the key issues. Relevant literature is integrated with current clinical and research information. This text should provide a quick, comprehensive review and valuable resource for current diagnosis and treatment.

Suggested management strategies are designed to assist the practitioner when addressing difficult headache problems, with special attention given to migraine and its variants in childhood and adolescence. Our approach to acute and preventive treatment with the introduction of migraine-specific medication is clearly and comprehensively reviewed. In addition, the text delineates key clinical symptoms to help differentiate secondary headache syndromes from primary headache syndromes (migraine), with suggested diagnostic strategies. We hope this text will help to improve your practice satisfaction as well as your patient's satisfaction as it relates to the management of headache.

We would like to thank the authors who contributed to this text; their devotion and contributions are most appreciated. This work would not have been possible without the instruction and guidance of our former and present professors—in particular, Isabelle Rapin, Alfred Spiro, Niko Moshe, Shlmo Schinnar, Seymour Solomon, Randy Peterson, Seymour Diamond, Sidney Carter, Arnold Gold, Abe Chutorian, Nils Low, and Robert Kunkle.

In addition, we are indebted to Jennifer Mallory, Sue Cooper, and the entire team at B C Decker Inc for their assistance in the preparation of this material.

Finally, we thank our families for always being so understanding—our parents for all their encouragement, our wives for their patience and support, and our children who inspire us.

Paul Winner

A. David Rothner

Introduction

Children and adolescents frequently have significant incapacitating headaches. In one study, 56% of boys and 74% of girls between the ages of 12 and 17 reported having experienced a headache within the past month. The vast majority of those who seek medical help will prove to have migraine with or without aura, a migraine subclassification, or other primary headache disorder. Cluster headache, one of the primary headache disorders, has been reported in children as young as 3 years, but it is rare under the age of 10 years and uncommon before age 20.

Parents seek medical attention for their child or adolescent with headache primarily to rule out a brain tumor or other serious medical condition. A small number of children and adolescents will require additional studies to rule out an ominous etiology. This text will address in detail the symptoms, signs, and criteria to help the practitioner outline an appropriate plan of evaluation and intervention.

Once a correct headache diagnosis is confirmed, then appropriate management options can be reviewed with the patient and parent. This is often an opportune time to briefly review the present state of knowledge regarding the etiology of headache.

The headache management options for adult patients have increased significantly in the past years. Many of these options are being studied for appropriate use in the pediatric population. Guidelines for treatment options, both pharmacologic and nonpharmacologic, for children and adolescents are addressed in this text.

The initial description of the sick headache dates back over 4,000 years. Hippocrates, in approximately 400 BC, described what appears to be migraine with aura. Very few references were made concerning the subject of headache in children until 1873 when William Henry Day, a British pediatrician, devoted a chapter to the subject of headache in children. He recognized that nonorganic, nonvascular headaches were most common in children. In 1962, Bille reported on the incidence and nature of headaches in over 9,000 school children. Friedman and Harms, in 1967, edited the first book on the subject of headache in children. In recent years, the number of works dealing with headache in children and adolescents has increased. This text is designed to help the practitioner address the unique differences regarding the diagnosis, evaluation, and treatment options posed by the presentation of headache in children and adolescents. Can we make a difference in children's lives by recognizing the etiology of their headaches and treating them appropriately? Yes!

Paul Winner

A. David Rothner

Chapter 1

EPIDEMIOLOGY AND CLASSIFICATION OF HEADACHE

Richard B. Lipton, Joseph Maytal, and Paul Winner

There is a high incidence, prevalence, and individual and societal cost of headache disorders in children and adolescents. Validating an appropriate system for their diagnosis and classification is an important priority for both clinical practice and clinical research. Various classification schemes have been proposed for headache disorders in adolescents and children. The criteria proposed by the International Headache Society (IHS) represent a seminal advance, although these criteria were developed primarily for headache disorders in adults.[1] A series of studies on the diagnosis of headache in children and adolescents provides an empiric basis for recommending revisions to the IHS criteria for migraine in these age groups.[2–7] Revised and emerging criteria provide an important tool for clinical practice, clinical trials, and epidemiologic research.

In the IHS system, the primary headache disorders (migraine, tension-type headache, and cluster headache) are defined based on the symptom profiles and on the pattern of headache attacks.[1,8] The general medical and neurologic examinations, as well as diagnostic tests, serve primarily to exclude secondary headaches. In the absence of a diagnostic "gold standard," clinicians and researchers have struggled to develop valid and reliable diagnostic criteria for these disorders. The lack of standardized case definitions has plagued epidemiologic studies of headache and has contributed to the enormous variation in estimates of the prevalence and incidence of primary headache disorders.[9–13] The fundamental interrelationships of the primary headache disorders remain controversial. Although the IHS criteria view migraine and tension-type headache as distinct disorders, they are sometimes regarded as polar ends on a continuum of severity.[1,14,15]

Other features of primary headache disorders complicate both clinical diagnosis and epidemiologic research. Migraine is a heterogeneous disorder; attacks vary in pain intensity, duration, pattern of associated features, and frequency of occurrence.[16–19] This lack of uniformity in disease manifestations among individuals complicates the development of highly sensitive and specific case definitions. Because migraine is an episodic disorder, its manifestations also vary within individuals over time.[16] Headaches may undergo exacerbations or remissions in children. Because both clinicians and epidemiologists must rely on the recall of patients or parents, diagnoses are subject to recall bias. The most severe, frequent, or dramatic attacks may be preferentially reported.[12] Many migraineurs have more than one headache type and may have trouble recalling which symptoms were associated with each headache type.[16]

Selection and referral bias have also limited progress in the epidemiologic study of migraine.[12] Most headache studies are conducted in samples derived from primary or specialty care settings. Many headache sufferers never seek care at all, and only a small percentage ever consult neurologists or headache specialists.[20,21] Consultation rates increase with age.[21] In clinic-based studies, factors that lead to consultation may be mistaken for attributes of the disease. For example, several clinic-based studies reported an association between migraine and high socioeconomic status (SES).[12] However, when this association was tested in a population-based survey, an inverse relationship between migraine and SES was identified: migraine is a disease of high SES in the clinic but not in the community.[8,22] These data suggest a referral bias in the clinic-based studies: migraineurs with high income are more likely to be referred to neurologists. Therefore, confirmation of findings from clinic-based studies in population-based samples is necessary. The problem of selection bias is partially circumvented in studies of pediatric headache due to the excellent school-based studies. Schools provide reasonably representative samples of children living in a particular area.[23–25]

DIAGNOSTIC CRITERIA
FOR PEDIATRIC MIGRAINE

Over the last three decades, several definitions of pediatric migraine have been proposed (Table 1–1). Vahlquist,[26] followed by Bille,[24] defined migraine as paroxysmal headaches separated by symptom-free intervals and accompanied by at least two of four of the following features: (1) unilaterality, (2) nausea, (3) visual aura, and (4) family history of migraine. In 1962, the Ad Hoc Committee on Classification of Headaches provided a description of migraine but did not specify which features had to be present to make a diagnosis.[27] Since that time, other researchers have proposed minor revisions to the Vahlquist criteria.[28]

In 1988, the IHS proposed a new set of criteria for migraine headaches based on international expert consensus (see Table 1–1).[1] The utility of the

Table 1–1   Definitions of Childhood Migraine

Lead Author/Year	Number of Attacks and Duration	Pain and Associated Features
Vahlquist[26] (1955)	Recurrent headaches with symptom-free intervals	At least two of nausea, visual aura, unilaterality, positive family history
Prensky and Sommer[28] (1979)	Recurrent headache separated by symptom-free intervals	At least three of nausea or vomiting, abdominal pain, aura, unilaterality, positive family history, throbbing or pulsatile pain
International Headache Society[1] (1988) Migraine without aura	At least five lifetime attacks Headache duration 2–48 hours if < 15 years old Headache duration 4–72 hours if ≥ 15 years old	One of two of photophobia *and* phonophobia, nausea or vomiting Two of four of unilateral pain, throbbing or pulsatile pain, moderate to severe intensity, exacerbation by routine physical activity
Winner et al.[30] (1996) IHS-Revised	At least five lifetime attacks lasting 1–48 hours	Two of four of bilateral (frontal/temporal) or unilateral, throbbing or pulsatile pain, moderate or severe intensity, exacerbation with routine physical activity One of two of photophobia *or* phonophobia, nausea or vomiting
Maytal et al.[4] (1997)	At least five lifetime attacks lasting 1–48 hours	One of three of unilaterality, throbbing pain, moderate or severe intensity One of four of nausea, vomiting, photophobia, or phonophobia

IHS criteria for pediatric headache disorders has been challenged primarily because expert clinical diagnosis and IHS-based diagnosis often disagree. Reported levels of agreement have ranged from 44 to 66%.[2–4,6,29,30] For example, Seshia et al. examined a specialty referral sample of 77 children (median age 11).[6] They found full agreement between clinical and IHS diagnosis in 44 children (61%), partial agreement in 22 children (31%), and complete lack of agreement in 6 children (8%). In a multicenter prospective study, Winner et al. reported full agreement in 58 children (66%).[30] In a similar referral sample, Maytal et al. found an overall level of agreement of 53%.[4] Using the clinical diagnosis as the gold standard, in several studies the sensitivity of the IHS criteria has ranged from 47 to 66%.[3,4,29–31] In Maytal et al., the specificity of the IHS criteria was 92.4%.[4]

The relatively modest sensitivity of the IHS criteria suggests that these criteria are more restrictive in comparison with expert clinical diagnosis. This may be problematic in clinical practice, where a clinician usually assigns a diagnosis as a prelude to treatment. There are other difficulties in applying strict criteria in childhood. In some children, prostration, nausea, repeated vomiting, and abdominal discomfort may overshadow the complaint of headache.[31] In addition, young children and their parents may not be able to describe the pain or the associated features of the attacks in the terms required by the IHS criteria. For example, in their specialty center-based study, Seshia et al. found that in children with headaches, 30% could not describe the quality of their pain and 16% could not report on photophobia and phonophobia.[6] Inability to report migraine-defining features may lead to underdiagnosis using strict IHS criteria.

The IHS-based diagnoses have also been compared with diagnoses assigned using other sets of criteria. Metsahonkala and Sillanpaa[32] compared the IHS definition of migraine with six other standard sets of criteria. In their sample, 95 children had IHS migraine, 106 had Vahlquist migraine, and 83 had both. In a multicenter prospective study, Winner et al. compared the IHS definition of migraine with a revised definition they termed IHS-R (see Table 1–1).[30] They reported that the IHS-R definition had higher sensitivity (93%) than the IHS definition (66%) using clinical diagnosis as the gold standard.[30] In an independent study, using clinical diagnosis as the gold standard,[29] Winner et al. reported that the IHS definition had a sensitivity of 53%, the Vahlquist definition had a sensitivity of

69%, and the IHS-R had a sensitivity of 80%. These studies show that the IHS criteria are more restrictive than the Vahlquist criteria, although there were bidirectional differences in classification.

In a subspecialty center study, Wober-Bingol et al. assessed 437 children and adolescents to identify 409 patients with primary headache disorders.[7] They included all seven IHS-defined migraine subtypes including IHS 1.7 (migrainous disorder not fulfilling the criteria). This category is used for patients who meet all of the IHS criteria for migraine but one. Of the 262 patients with migraine in their sample, 84 (32%) were in the IHS 1.7 category. The authors suggest that the IHS criteria should be revised to increase the proportion of clinically diagnosed migraineurs classified as full IHS migraine without resorting to the IHS 1.7 group.

Using a different approach, several authors have assessed the diagnostic utility of individual IHS-defining features of migraine. In children and adolescents, migraine tends to be of shorter duration. The IHS criteria take this into account by permitting shorter headache duration for patients under age 15 years (2 to 48 hours) than for those over 15 years (4 to 72 hours).[1] Of those with a clinical diagnosis of migraine, from 11 to 81% have a headache duration of less than 2 hours and from 8 to 25% have a headache duration of less than 1 hour.[2–4,29,30] Several investigators have therefore argued that the minimum duration required for diagnosis should be reduced from 2 hours to 1 hour. Winner et al. reported that making this reduction increased the diagnostic sensitivity from 66 to 78% using clinical diagnosis as the gold standard.[30] The authors support the suggestion to decrease the minimal duration requirement to 1 hour.[4] Maytal et al. showed that decreasing the minimal duration to less than 1 hour produced small gains in the sensitivity but substantially reduced the specificity of the definition in one study.[4]

Unilateral pain has been challenged as a diagnostic criterion because it is more characteristic of adult migraine than of pediatric migraine.[2,3,7,29,30] For example, Metsahonkala and Sillanpaa[32] reported that 67% of their migraineurs had unilateral pain. Gallai et al. found that 41.5% of their IHS migraineurs had unilateral pain.[2] Maytal et al. found that unilateral pain had a sensitivity of 34% and a specificity of 86% using clinical diagnosis as the gold standard.[4] Although bilateral headache is common in children, unilaterality has a high positive predictive value for migraine of 85%.[4] For this reason, Maytal et al. argue that unilateral pain should remain a migraine-defining feature in children (see Table 1–1).[4] The limitation in sensitivity is offset in the current IHS criteria by making it one of several alternative pain features.

Other migraine characteristics such as pain intensity and pulsatile quality of pain are sometimes difficult to ascertain in pediatric patients. In a series of studies, throbbing or pulsatile pain had a sensitivity of 36 to 86%.[2,4,7,25,32] Similarly, the sensitivity of moderate to severe intensity varied from 57.8 to 97.1%.[2,4–11,25] We believe that these pain features should remain part of the IHS definition in children as long as they are accurately ascertained. Associated symptoms such as nausea, vomiting, and photophobia had good sensitivity.[4,6,32] As part of their IHS-R criteria, Winner et al. noted that if photophobia *or* phonophobia, rather than photophobia *and* phonophobia, is used, sensitivity improves, especially in the subset under 12 years of age.[29] Phonophobia with or without photophobia was deemed important because of its high specificity and positive predictive value; its low sensitivity can be offset by using it as one of several alternative features.[4] Several authors have included family history as part of the case definition.[6,26] We recommend against this because informant histories of migraine are often inaccurate; in addition, because migraine is very common, it may occur in families by coincidence.[33]

Maytal et al. explored several alternative symptom-based case definitions using clinical diagnosis as the gold standard.[4] Eliminating the requirement for a minimal headache duration improved sensitivity but substantially decreased specificity. The case definition that optimized sensitivity and specificity required five headache attacks, duration of 1 to 48 hours, one of three pain features (unilaterality, throbbing, moderate or severe pain intensity), and one of four associated features (nausea, vomiting, photophobia, or phonophobia). Using the clinician's diagnosis as the gold standard, this case definition for migraine without aura had a sensitivity of 71.6% and a specificity of 70.9%. Thus, even the optimal case definition did not simultaneously provide high sensitivity and specificity relative to a clinical gold standard.

Several factors may account for the difficulty in improving agreement between clinical and criteria-based diagnosis of pediatric migraine. First, diagnosticians may rely on features of migraine (such as osmophobia or pallor) that are not included in the current diagnostic criteria. Further, children with migraine sometimes have atypical presentations including recurrent episodes of abdominal pain or vertigo with or without headache. Research criteria do not capture these features. In addition, young children and their parents may not be able to describe the pain or the associated features of the attacks in the terms required by the IHS criteria.

As our understanding of migraine evolves, the case definition of migraine both for children and adults is likely to change. In the absence of a true gold standard, diagnostic validity must be approached by searching for convergent evidence.[10,11] If we make the criteria for migraine very "loose," sensitivity will be optimized at the price of specificity. If we make criteria more restrictive, specificity will be optimized at the price of sensitivity. The appropriate balance between sensitivity and specificity depends on the diagnostician's objectives. For clinical practice, it is not practical to have a large undiagnosed group. For research, diagnosing nonmigraineurs with migraine may substantially attenuate efforts to identify genetic or biologic markers as well as treatment effects; in this context, specificity is critical. Future work should focus on alternative case definitions based on behavior rather than symptoms (i.e., going to a dark room, squinting, turning off the lights instead of photophobia). Exploring additional or alternative diagnostic features (e.g., pallor, abdominal pain, sensitivity to odors, menstrual exacerbation) may be helpful. For clinical trials, beyond case definition, inclusion and exclusion criteria can be used to ensure that patient selection corresponds to the research objectives.

In epidemiologic research, variation in the case definition will influence estimates of incidence and prevalence. While the case definition emerges, the IHS criteria remain the best available gold standard. In the next sections, we consider the available data on the epidemiology of pediatric migraine.

MIGRAINE INCIDENCE

Incidence refers to the rate of onset of new cases of a particular disease in a defined population. Few prospective studies have addressed the age-specific incidence of migraine in population-based samples, in part because estimating the incidence of episodic disorders poses unique challenges.[34] In a population-based study, Stewart et al.[35] estimated migraine incidence using reported age of migraine onset. Telescoping, the tendency to report the time of events in the past at a time closer to the present, limits the accuracy of these estimates.[36] In addition, someone with migraine in the distant past may forget that he or she had attacks or forget the features of the attack. Stewart et al. used a mathematic model to adjust for telescoping. They also used a case definition that minimized the effects of unreliable reporting.[35]

They conducted telephone interviews in over 10,000 individuals aged 12 to 29 years. Age- and gender-specific incidence rates for migraine with and without aura were estimated based on 392 males and 1,018 females with migraine. The incidence of migraine was lower in males than females and occurred at an earlier age. The incidence of migraine with aura in males was 6.6 per 1,000 person-years and peaked at 5 to 6 years of age. The peak incidence of migraine without aura in males was 10 per 1,000 person-years and peaked between the ages of 10 and 11 years. New cases of migraine were uncommon in men in their twenties. For females, the incidence of migraine with aura was 14.1 per 1,000 person-years with a peak at ages 12 to 13 years; the incidence of migraine without aura was 18.9 per 1,000 person-years and peaked at ages 14 to 17. Because of the restricted age range of this study, data concerning children under 12 years or adults over 29 years cannot be provided.

Stang et al.[37] used very different methods to study migraine incidence. They used the linked medical records system in Olmstead County, Minnesota, to identify new cases of migraine. Medical records were reviewed to establish the type and age of onset of headache. No distinction was made between migraine with and without aura. Age-specific incidence was lower in Rochester, Minnesota, than in the study by Stewart et al.[35] because many people with migraine do not consult doctors for headache.[21] Stang et al. also found incidence peaks later than those reported by Stewart et al., in part because medical consultation occurs well after onset of migraine in some people.[21,37]

The linked medical records system provides excellent epidemiologic data for conditions that are completely ascertained by the health care system. Under-ascertainment of headaches is very likely using this method. In addition, very early-onset cases (e.g., < 6 years of age) may not be effectively diagnosed because of the difficulties very young patients have in articulating their symptoms. If these early-onset cases are less likely to be ascertained, the median age of onset will be overestimated. Although these are limitations, Stang et al. provide useful data on incidence and patterns of medical consultation.

MIGRAINE PREVALENCE

Table 1–2 summarizes a number of school- and population-based studies that have examined the prevalence of headache in children. By age 3 years, headache occurs in 3 to 8% of children.[38–40] At age 5, 19.5% have headache, and by age 7, 37 to 51.5% have headache.[24,41–43] In 7 to 15 year olds, headache prevalence ranges from 57 to 82%.[24,41–43] Mortimer et al. showed increases in headache prevalence from ages 3 to 11 in both boys and girls with higher headache prevalence in 3- to 5-year-old boys than in 3- to 5-year-old girls (Table 1–3).[5] Thus, the overall prevalence of headache increases quite strikingly from preschool-age children to midadolescence when examined using various cross-sectional studies.

Sillanpaa et al.[41,42,44] conducted a longitudinal study in a school-based sample of 1,205 children evaluated at ages 7, 14, 15, 16, and 22. As Table 1–4 shows, headache prevalence in boys was stable from ages 7 to 14 and declined thereafter. Girls showed modest increases in headache prevalence from ages 7 to 22. The differences between these longitudinal results and prior reports in cross-sectional studies are not well understood. Aromaa et al.[45] investigated the predictors of childhood headaches in 1,443 families and found that the mother's assessment of the infant's poor health and feeding problems were strong headache predictors at the age of 9 months, whereas depression and sleeping difficulties were strong predictors at 3 years of age.

The prevalence of migraine varies with case definition;[13] studies using the IHS criteria have yielded surprisingly uniform results.[14,17,22,46–48] A number of studies have specifically examined migraine prevalence in pediatric age groups (see Table 1–2). Migraine prevalence at age 7 ranges from 1.2 to 3.2%.[5,24,38] By ages 7 to 15, prevalence ranges from 4 to 11%.[5,24,38,39] In one of the best contemporary studies, Mortimer et al. directly interviewed 1,083 children (ages 3 to 11 years) registered with a United Kingdom general practice.[5] Of 1,104 eligible children, 1,083 (98.1%) participated in a

Table 1–2 Prevalence of Headache and Migraine by Age in Selected Community and School-Based Studies

Lead Author (Year) Country	Type of Population	Sample Size	Age Range (Years)	Time Frame	Migraine Definition	Headache Prevalence			Migraine Prevalence		
						Males	Females	Overall	Males	Females	Overall
Abu-Arafeh[23] (1994), UK	School children	1,754	5–15	1 year	IHS*	—	—	—	—	—	10.6
Bille[24] (1962), Sweden	School children	8,993	7–15	Lifetime	Vahlquist*	58.0	59.3	—	3.3	4.4	—
Linet[12] (1984), USA	Community	10,132	12–29	1 year	Two of NV/U/VA	90	95	—	5.3	14	—
Mortimer[5] (1992), UK	General practice	1,083	3–11	1 year	IHS*	40.6	36.9	38.8	4.1	2.9	3.7
Raieli[25] (1995), Italy	School children	1,445	11–14	1 year	IHS*	19.9	28.0	23.9	2.7	3.3	3.0
Sillanpaa[38] (1976), Finland	School children	4,825	3	?	Vahlquist*	—	—	—	—	—	—
			7	?		—	4.3	—	3.2	3.2	3.2
Sillanpaa[41] (1983), Finland	School children	3,784	13	1 year	Vahlquist*	79.8	84.2	—	8.1	15.1	—
Zuckerman[40] (1987), UK	Consecutive births	308	3	1 month	—	—	4	—	—	—	—

IHS = International Headache Society; N = nausea; U = unilateral; V = vomiting; VA = visual aura.
*See Table 1–1.

Table 1–3   One-Year Prevalence of
Headache and IHS Migraine in School Children

Age Groups (Years)	Headache (Last Year)		IHS Migraine (Last Year)	
	Boys	Girls	Boys	Girls
3–5	26.4	17.5	1.9	1.0
5–7	36.4	35.0	4.3	1.2
7–9	44.5	43.5	4.7	4.8
9–11	54.9	51.6	6.2	6.4

IHS = International Headache Society.
Adapted from: Mortimer J, Kay J, Jaron A. Epidemiology of headache and childhood migraine in an urban general practice using Ad Hoc, Vahlquist and IHS criteria. Dev Med Child Neurol 1992;34:1095–1101.

"structured interview." Subjects with possible migraine took part in an extended interview designed to assess three sets of migraine diagnostic criteria: Vahlquist, Ad Hoc, and IHS (see Table 1–1 for definitions). As Table 1–3 shows, IHS migraine prevalence was higher in boys than girls at ages 3 to 5 and 5 to 7. In 7 to 11 year olds, prevalence is equivalent in boys and girls.

Mortimer et al. also explored the variation in migraine prevalence by case definition.[5] As Table 1–5 shows, there was little variation by case definition for the migraine with aura group. However, for migraine without aura, prevalence was lowest using the IHS definition, 23% higher using the Vahlquist definition, and over 50% higher using the Ad Hoc definition. This within-study exploration is consistent with the meta-analytic result across studies; estimates of migraine prevalence vary strikingly with case definition.[13]

Table 1–4   Prevalence of Headache by Age and Gender
in 1,205 Children During 15 Years of Follow-Up

Age (Years)	Headache Prevalence		Migraine Prevalence		Total
	Boys	Girls	Boys	Girls	
7	50.5	49.5	2.9	2.5	2.7
14	48.6	51.4	6.4	14.8	10.6
22	36.5	63.5	—	—	—

Adapted from: Sillanpaa M. Headache in children. In: Oleson J, ed. Headache Classification and Epidemiology. New York: Raven Press, 1994, pp 273–281; and Sillanpaa M. Changes in the prevalence of migraine and other headaches during the first seven school years. Headache 1983;23:15–19.

Table 1–5   Prevalence of Migraine by Diagnostic Criteria in School Children

Criteria	Migraine without Aura (%)	Migraine with Aura (%)	Total (%)
Vahlquist	2.7	1.5	4.2
Ad Hoc	3.4	1.5	4.9
International Headache Society	2.2	1.5	3.7

Adapted from: Mortimer J, Kay J, Jaron A. Epidemiology of headache and childhood migraine in an urban general practice using Ad Hoc, Vahlquist and IHS criteria. Dev Med Child Neurol 1992;34:1095–1101.

Raieli et al. assessed the prevalence of migraine headache in an epidemiologic survey of 11- to 14-year-old students.[25] A population registry for the municipality of Monreale, Italy, provided the sampling frame. Students were interviewed by neurologists at school using semistructured interviews. The authors found that headache prevalence increased uniformly in girls but appeared stable in boys. Overall migraine prevalence was 3.0% with a slight female preponderance. It is not clear why the estimates of Raieli et al. are lower than those of other studies in this age group.

The age-prevalence profile in adolescents and adults was explored in the American Migraine Study. In that study, there is a monotonic increase in migraine prevalence in both males and females from age 12 to about age 40.[22] After midlife, prevalence declined. This study also reported that the female to male gender ratio increases from age 12 to about age 42, after which time it declines.[22] The decline in gender ratio after age 42 corresponds in time with declining estrogen levels as menopause approaches.[49] This pattern suggests that hormonal or neural events associated with menarche may contribute to the emerging relative increases in the prevalence of migraine in females in early adolescence.

Several studies, including one that focuses on children, suggest that migraine prevalence may be increasing.[37,50,51] An analysis of data from the National Health Interview Study (NHIS) showed that migraine prevalence increased 60% from 25.8 per 1,000 population to 41 per 1,000 population between 1981 and 1989.[50] Using a linked medical records system, an increase in prevalence was observed in Rochester, Minnesota, even before 1981.[37] The NHIS diagnosed migraine based on self-report. In Rochester, Minnesota, only medically ascertained headache cases were identified.

Increases in migraine awareness, consultation rates, and diagnosis could account for these provocative results without a true increase in prevalence.

A study from Finland provides more compelling evidence that the prevalence of both headache and migraine is increasing in children. Sillanpaa and Antilla conducted two identical cross-sectional studies of migraine prevalence in school children in 1974 and again in 1992.[51] Each study examined 7 year olds using the same nine-item screening questionnaires. In 1974, the prevalence of migraine in 7 year olds was 1.9%; in 1992, it had increased to 5.7%. Increases occurred in both boys and girls, suggesting that the secular trends described in the United States[37,50] also pertain to children in Finland. If these secular trends in prevalence are confirmed, it is important to identify the factors that have caused these prevalence increases.

What could account for the increasing prevalence of migraine and headache? Since the magnitude of the increase was comparable for migraine and for headache, it is parsimonious to search for a common explanation for both findings. A putative cause would presumably have to influence both children and adults in the United States and Finland. Sillanpaa and Antilla[51] suggest that changes in the social environment may play a role. Other widely distributed environmental risk factors such as food additives could account for these results. Although the causes are not clear, given the enormous burden of headache, these findings mandate additional studies. Future studies should use systematic samples with rigorous application of diagnostic criteria to clarify the magnitude, distribution, and etiology of these prevalence increases.

Longitudinal data on migraine outcome from unselected samples are relatively sparse. Bille followed a sample of children with severe migraine for periods of up to 37 years; although remissions of up to 2 years were frequent, after 30 years only 40% continued to be migraine free.[24,52,53] These data suggest that migraine may be a lifelong disorder with prolonged remissions in many people. Hockaday noted long-term remissions: cessation of migraine in 35% of male and 21% of female migraineurs after an interval of 8 to 25 years.[31]

Congdon and Forsythe in a follow-up of 300 children aged 5 to 14 years found that 29% had an 8-year remission and 34% had a 10-year remission.[54] In a Mayo Clinic study, 9 to 14 years after treatment, 32.8%

were completely free of headache and 46.6% considerably improved.[55] Bille investigated how frequently migraine recurs in adult life.[53] He reported that of the original 73 patients in his study with "more pronounced migraine," after 23 years, 60% were still having migraine attacks. A large number had been free for several years. The evolution of headaches in childhood and adolescence was evaluated recently by Guidetti and Galli[56] in an 8-year follow-up study. They noted that the overall remission rate of headaches was 34%; worsening was noted in 6%, and the condition remained unchanged in 15%. Additional longitudinal data from population-based studies are required to clarify the natural history of migraine.

Sillanpaa followed a cohort of 2,921 school children from age 7 to age 22 and examined migraine outcome as a function of age of onset (Table 1–6).[38] Of migraineurs with onset prior to age 7, 26% of boys and 19% of girls had a total remission of headache. Thus, boys were more likely than girls to experience a complete remission. About one-third of each group had a partial remission. For the group with headache onset between the ages of 8 and 14, 22% of boys and 27% of girls experienced a complete remission.

Studies from specialty clinics suggest that there is a subgroup of adult migraine sufferers afflicted with a progressive syndrome termed "transformed migraine."[57,58] With this condition, attacks increase in frequency over a number of years until a pattern of daily or near-daily headache evolves.[57–61] In samples from subspecialty clinics, this disorder is associated with overuse of acute headache medications. Medication overuse is also believed to contribute to the accelerating pattern of pain through a mechanism that has

Table 1–6   Dynamics of Migraine in a Cohort of
2,921 School Children Followed for Up to 15 Years

Age of Onset (Years)	Outcome	Proportion of Subjects with Outcome at Age 22	
		Boys	Girls
≤ 7	Total remission	26	19
	Partial remission	37	37
	Persistent	37	44
8–14	Total remission	22	27
	Persistent	78	73

Adapted from: Sillanpaa M. Headache in children. In: Olesen J, ed. Headache Classification and Epidemiology. New York: Raven Press, 1994, pp 273–281.

been termed "rebound headache." When the cycle of medication overuse is broken, headaches often improve.[57–61] However, in subspecialty clinics, this process of acceleration occurs in the absence of medication overuse in about 20% of patients, suggesting that there is a subgroup of migraine sufferers with a progressive condition.[57,58] Transformed migraine occurs in about 1.3% in population samples.[62] Population-based case-control and cohort studies are needed to fully assess the influence of appropriate and inappropriate treatment patterns and other risk factors on the development of transformed migraine. Perhaps patient education and early aggressive treatment combined with avoidance of medication overuse in children and adolescents could reduce the risk of transformed chronic migraine.

CONCLUSION

The development of the IHS criteria provided a uniform case definition for migraine that has greatly facilitated epidemiologic and biologic headache research as well as clinical trials. Although an IHS-based diagnosis of migraine is conservative (in that many children and adolescents with a clinical diagnosis of migraine do not meet IHS criteria), this approach identifies a relatively homogeneous group of patients. Therefore, it provides a firm basis for clinical trials in children and adolescents. In clinical practice, an excessively restrictive case definition is problematic in that many individuals with the disease may not be diagnosed. In epidemiologic research, an excessively restrictive case definition of migraine in children will lead to underestimation of the prevalence. For biologic research, which contrasts migraine cases and controls, a restrictive case definition may lead to inclusion of individuals who actually have migraine in the control group. This type of misclassification will lead to underestimation of the association between a biologic or genetic marker and migraine.

Despite the concerns about the case definition of migraine in children and adolescents, this has been a time of enormous progress in migraine research. As issues about the case definition are debated, additional longitudinal studies are required to better define the natural history of migraine and the risk factors for disease progression. As pathogenic genes are discovered, exploration of the relationships between genotypes and phenotypes as well as gene-environment interactions may help clarify issues of classification and risk. Additional efforts to measure disease burden on children and adolescents as well as their families will complement similar efforts that have already been undertaken in adults with migraine.

REFERENCES

1. Classification and diagnostic criteria for headache disorders, cranial neuralgias and facial pain. Headache Classification Committee of the International Headache Society. Cephalalgia 1988;8(Suppl 7):1–96.

2. Gallai V, Sarchielli P, Carboni F, et al Applicability of the 1988 IHS criteria to headache patients under the age of 18 years attending 21 Italian headache clinics. Headache 1995;35:146–153.

3. Gladstein J, Holden EW, Perotta L, Raven M. Diagnosis and symptom patterns in children presenting to a pediatric headache clinic. Headache 1993;33:497–500.

4. Maytal J, Young M, Schechter A, Lipton RB. Pediatric migraine and the International Headache Society (IHS) criteria. Neurology 1997;48:602–607.

5. Mortimer J, Kay J, Jaron A. Epidemiology of headache and childhood migraine in an urban general practice using Ad Hoc, Vahlquist and IHS criteria. Dev Med Child Neurol 1992;34:1095–1101.

6. Seshia S, Wolstein J, Adams C, et al International Headache Society criteria and childhood headache. Dev Med Child Neurol 1994;36:419–428.

7. Wober-Bingol C, Wober C, Karwautz A, et al Diagnosis of headache in childhood and adolescence: a study in 437 patients. Cephalalgia 1995;15:13–21.

8. Lipton RB, Stewart WF. Prevalence and impact of migraine. Neurol Clin 1997;15:1–13.

9. Lipton RB, Stewart WF, Merikangas K. Reliability in headache diagnosis. Cephalalgia 1993;13(Suppl 12):29–33.

10. Merikangas KR, Angst J, Isler H. Migraine and psychopathology: results of the Zurich cohort study of young adults. Arch Gen Psychiatry 1990;47:849–853.

11. Merikangas KR, Frances A. Development of diagnostic criteria for headache syndromes: lessons from psychiatry. Cephalalgia 1993;13(Suppl 12):34–38.

12. Linet MS. Stewart WF. Migraine headache: epidemiologic perspectives. Epidemiol Rev 1984;6:107–139.

13. Stewart WF, Simon D, Schechter A, Lipton RB. Population variation in migraine prevalence: a meta-analysis. J Clin Epidemiol 1995;48:269–280.

14. Featherstone HJ. Migraine and muscle contraction headaches: a continuum. Headache 1985;24:194–198.

15. Raskin NH. Headache. 2nd ed. New York: Churchill-Livingston, 1988.

16. Johannes CB, Linet MS, Stewart WF, et al. Relationship of headache to phase of the menstrual cycle among young women: a daily diary study. Neurology 1995;45:1076–1082.

17. Rasmussen BK, Jensen R, Schroll M, Olesen J. Epidemiology of headache in a general population—a prevalence study. J Clin Epidemiol 1991;44:1147–1157.

18. Rasmussen BK, Olesen J. Migraine with aura and migraine without aura. An epidemiologic study. Cephalalgia 1992;12:229–237.

19. Stewart WF, Schechter A, Lipton RB. Migraine heterogeneity: disability, pain intensity, and attack frequency and duration. Neurology 1994;44 (Suppl 6):24–39.

20. Lipton RB, Stewart WF, Celentano DD, Reed ML. Undiagnosed migraine: a comparison of symptom-based and self-reported physician diagnosis. Arch Intern Med 1992;152:1273–1278.

21. Lipton RB, Stewart WF, Simon D. Medical consultation for migraine: results from the American Migraine Study. Headache 1998;38(2):87–96.

22. Stewart WF, Lipton RB, Celentano DD, Reed ML. Prevalence of migraine headache in the United States. JAMA 1992;267:64–69.

23. Abu-Arefeh I, Russell G. Prevalence of headache and migraine in school children. BMJ 1994;309:765–769.

24. Bille B. Migraine in school children. Acta Paediatr Scand 1962;51(Suppl 136): 1–151.

25. Raieli V, Raimondo D, Cammalleri R, Camarda R. Migraine headache in adolescents: a student population-based study in Monreale. Cephalalgia 1995;15:5–12.

26. Vahlquist B. Migraine in children. Int Arch Allergy 1955;7:348–352.

27. Friedman AP, Finley KH, Graham JR. Classification of headache. Arch Neurol 1962;6:173–176.

28. Prensky AL, Sommer D. Diagnosis and treatment of migraine in children. Neurology 1979;29:506–510.

29. Winner P, Martinez W, Mante L, Bello L. Classification of pediatric migraine: proposed revisions to the IHS criteria. Headache 1995;35:407–410.

30. Winner P, Gladstein J, Hamel R, et al. Multicenter prospective evaluation of proposed pediatric migraine revisions to the IHS criteria. Presented at the American Association for the Study of Headache Scientific Meeting; San Diego, CA, May 1996.

31. Hockaday JM. Definitions, clinical features and diagnosis of childhood migraine. In: Hockaday JM, ed. Migraine in Children. London: Butterworth, 1988, pp 5–24.

32. Metsahonkala L, Sillanpaa M. Migraine in children: an evaluation of the IHS criteria. Cephalalgia 1994;14:285–290.

33. Ottman R, Hong S, Lipton RB. Validity of family history data on severe headache and migraine. Neurology 1993;43:1954–1960.

34. Cummings RG, Kelsey JL, Nevitt MC. Methodologic issues in the study of frequent and recurrent health problems. Ann Epidemiol 1990;1:49–56.

35. Stewart WF, Linet MS, Celentano DD, et al. Age- and sex-specific incidence rates of migraine with and without visual aura. Am J Epidemiol 1993; 34:1111–1120.

36. Brown NR, Rips LJ, Shevelle SK. The subjective dates of natural events in very long term memory. Cogn Psychol 1985;17:139–177.

37. Stang PE, Yanagihara T, Swanson JW, et al Incidence of migraine headaches: a population-based study in Olmstead County, Minnesota. Neurology 1992;42:1657–1662.

38. Sillanpaa M. Prevalence of migraine and other headache in Finnish children starting school. Headache 1976;15:288–290.

39. Sillanpaa M. Headache in children. In: Olesen J, ed. Headache Classification and Epidemiology. New York: Raven Press, 1994, pp 273–281.

40. Zuckerman B, Stevenson J, Bailey V. Stomachaches and headaches in a community sample of preschool children. Pediatrics 1987;79:677–682.

41. Sillanpaa M. Changes in the prevalence of migraine and other headaches during the first seven school years. Headache 1983;23:15–19.

42. Sillanpaa M, Piekkala P. Prevalence of migraine and other headaches in early puberty. Scand J Prim Health Care 1984;2:27–32.

43. Sillanpaa M, Piekkala P, Kero P. Prevalence of headache at preschool age in an unselected child population. Cephalalgia 1991;11:239–242.

44. Sillanpaa M. Prevalence of headache in prepuberty. Headache 1983;23: 10–14.

45. Aromaa M, Rautava P, Helenius H, Sillanpaa M. Factors of early life as predictors of headaches in children at school entry. Headache 1998;38:23–30.

46. Gobels H, Petersen-Braun M, Soyka D. The epidemiology of headache in Germany: a nationwide survey of a representative sample on the basis of the headache classification of the International Headache Society. Cephalalgia 1994;14:97–106.

47. Henry P, Michel P, Brochet B, et al. A nationwide survey of migraine in France: prevalence and clinical features in adults. Cephalalgia 1992; 12:229–237.

48. Pryse-Phillips W, Findlay H, Tugwell P, et al. A Canadian population survey on the clinical epidemiologic and societal impact of migraine and tension-type headache. Can J Neurol Sci 1992;19:333–339.

49. Silberstein SD. The role of sex hormones in headache. Neurology 1992; 42(Suppl 2):37–42.

50. U.S. Department of Health and Human Services/Public Health Services. Prevalence of chronic migraine headaches in the United States, 1980–1989. MMWR Morb Mortal Wkly Rep 1991;40:331,337–338.

51. Sillanpaa M, Antilla P. Increasing prevalence of headache in 7-year-old school children. Headache 1996;36:466–470.

52. Bille B. Migraine in childhood and its prognosis. Cephalalgia 1981;1:71–75.

53. Bille B. Migraine in children: prevalence, clinical features, and a 30-year follow up. In: Ferrari MD, Lataste X, eds. Migraine and Other Headaches. New Jersey: Parthenon, 1989.

54. Congdon PJ, Forsythe WI. Migraine in childhood: a study of 300 children. Dev Med Child Neurol 1979;21:209–216.

55. Hinrichs WL, Keith HM. Migraine in childhood: follow-up report. Mayo Clin Proc 1965;40:593–596.

56. Guidetti V, Galli F. Evolution of headache in childhood and adolescence: an 8-year follow-up. Cephalalgia 1998;18:449–454.

57. Mathew NT, Reuveni U, Perez F. Transformed or evolutive migraine. Headache 1987;27:102–106.

58. Mathew NT, Stubits E, Nigam MP. Transformation of episodic migraine into daily headache: analysis of factors. Headache 1982;22:66–68.

59. Raskin NH. Repetitive intravenous dihydroergotamine as therapy for intractable migraine. Neurology 1986;36:995–999.

60. Silberstein SD, Silberstein JR. Chronic daily headache: long-term prognosis following inpatient treatment with repetitive IV DHE. Headache 1992; 32:439–445.

61. Silberstein S, Lipton RB, Sliwinski M. Classification of daily and near-daily headache: a field study of revised IHS criteria. Neurology 1996;47:871–875.

62. Scher AL, Stewart WF, Liberman J, Lipton RB. Prevalence of frequent headache in a population sample. Submitted for publication, 1997.

Chapter 2

EVALUATION OF HEADACHE

A. David Rothner

A thorough evaluation of headache in children and adolescents is necessary to make the correct diagnosis and initiate treatment. The evaluation should include a detailed history and general and neurologic examinations. Based on this information, the differential diagnosis should be formulated identifying the type of headache and its likely etiology. Laboratory tests then may be needed to confirm the diagnosis or to rule out life-threatening etiologies. The next step is to monitor the clinical course to ensure the appropriate treatment, absence of side effects, and a favorable clinical course.

The evaluative process varies depending on the age of the child, headache acuity, severity of illness, and the need for intervention.

HISTORY

The history determines the correct diagnosis,[1,2] so questions need to be directed to both the child and parents (Table 2–1). Although computerized questionnaires have been used successfully, face-to-face dialogue is more valuable.[3] Children can provide useful information if questions are phrased appropriately. It is best to obtain a private interview with the adolescent patient. The physician should also note the interaction between patient and parents as it often reflects problems and conflicts not directly discussed.

Younger children react to pain by crying, rocking, and hiding.[4] When pain is chronic, regression, anxiety, and depression occur. Chronic pain impacts eating, sleeping, and playing. Emotional, behavioral, and personality factors assume even more importance as the child becomes an adolescent.

The history assesses the headache and its course over time (Figures 2–1 and 2–2). A headache diary or database can be quite useful.[5] Symptoms of increased intracranial pressure or progressive neurologic dysfunction should be noted, along with the family history and past medical history, including growth and development, a review of systems, injuries, operations, hospitalizations, serious illnesses, allergies, medications, drug reactions, alcohol or drug abuse, and educational and psychosocial status.

The Database

The headache database should include the following questions, as summarized in Table 2–1:

Table 2–1   Headache Database[6,7]

(1) Do you have one or more types of headache?

Some patients have more than one type of headache. It is important to establish the number of different headaches the patient has and to ask questions concerning each type separately. The physician needs to determine if the patient's headaches are all similar or if one is more severe (e.g., an adolescent patient who identifies mild daily headaches with superimposed severe headaches associated with nausea and vomiting twice monthly).

(2) How did the headaches begin?

Some patients can identify factors that may initiate the headaches. They may be physical (i.e., head trauma) or psychologic (e.g., parental separation, the death of a close relative or friend, a move to another community).

(3) When did the headaches begin?

Whether the headaches have been present for days, weeks, months, or years needs to be documented. In younger children, the parents will supply this information. The longer the headache has been present without symptoms of increased intracranial pressure or progressive neurologic signs the less likely it is an organic process. Migraine frequently has its onset in the first decade of life, whereas daily nonprogressive headaches begin in adolescence.

(4) Are the headaches intermittent, progressive, or staying the same?

The temporal pattern of each headache needs to be established (see Figures 2–1 and 2–2).[8] If the headache is new, rapidly becoming more severe, or associated with neurologic symptoms and signs, an organic process should be suspected. Intermittent headaches that occur one or two times per month and are associated with nausea and vomiting are most likely migraine. Headaches that occur daily or almost daily, last all day, and have been present for months without associated neurologic symptoms or signs are most likely a tension-type headache.

(5) How often does each headache type occur?

The headache frequency helps establish the type of headache. Migraine headaches usually occur two to four times per month. They never occur daily! Cluster headaches occur two to three times per day for weeks to months then disappear for months to years. Chronic nonprogressive headaches may occur daily for 5 to 7 days each week for months to years. The changing frequency of an established headache pattern may be significant.

Table 2–1 continued

(6) How long do the headaches last?

The duration is a clue to the headache type. Cluster and chronic paroxysmal hemicrania characteristically last 30 to 60 minutes. Migraine in younger children may be 1 hour or less and somewhat longer in adolescents. The discomfort of chronic muscle contraction headache may be continuous.

(7) Do the headaches occur at any special time or under any special circumstances?

The specific circumstances that cause the headaches need to be identified. Travel may precipitate migraine and school may be related to tension headaches, as may stress at home. Headache pain that awakens a child at night is of particular concern.

(8) Are the headaches related to specific foods, medications, or activities?

A small number of patients identify specific foods that provoke migraine. Headaches may occur with stimulants for attention deficit disorder (ADD) or with birth control pills. Overheating or exertion also may be causative. Headaches that occur or worsen with straining are ominous.

(9) Are there warning symptoms?

The young child can identify that something happens 10 to 15 minutes before the headache. The something may be a small headache that builds up into a big headache, blurred vision, or a feeling of warmth all over. Artistic children can be encouraged to draw their prodrome.[9] This question is frequently answered in the affirmative by the mother who notes that the child becomes quiet and pale and develops dark circles under the eyes. If the warning symptoms are persistently and repeatedly localized to the same side of the body, a seizure or structural etiology should be suspected.

(10) Where is the pain located?

The location of the pain may be specific or nonspecific. For example, the pain of otitis media is localized to one ear, that of optic neuritis and/or glaucoma and/or cluster headache to one eye, and that of temporomandibular joint disorder to the ipsilateral jaw. Young patients with migraine will describe bifrontal or bitemporal pain. Maxillary sinusitis is frequently localized to the face or eyes, whereas sphenoid sinusitis may cause vertex pain. The pain of cluster headaches and chronic paroxysmal hemicrania remains unilateral. Muscle contraction headaches cause bifrontal or bitemporal pain, which is described as band-like. Occipital headaches may be caused by basilar artery migraine, occipital neuralgia, or a craniocervical lesion such as the Arnold-Chiari malformation.

(11) What is the quality of the pain?

Many systems are used to measure children's pain, including facial drawings, a thermometer, or a numeric system.[10,11] Migraine is more severe than chronic nonprogressive headaches. When the patient describes the pain as being 10 out of 10 and shows no evidence of discomfort, stress-related headaches should be suspected.

(12) Are there associated symptoms during the headaches?

The examiner should question the presence of pallor, chills, flushing, fever, dizziness, syncope, behavioral changes, anorexia, abdominal pain, nausea, or vomiting. Aphasia, confusion, hemiparesis, vertigo, ophthalmoplegia. or loss of consciousness may rarely occur. If the headache is associated with neurologic symptoms or signs, an organic etiology should be sought.

Table 2–1 continued

(13) What do you do during your headaches?

What happens if the patients are at school? Do they seek medication or "tough it out." Do they lay their heads down or ask to go home? Nausea and vomiting usually require a visit to the nurse's office. If the children continue to play, the headache is usually not "serious." Children with migraine seek a dark, quiet place. Some adolescents with severe, chronic nonprogressive headaches are unable to attend school.

(14) What makes the headaches better?

Lying quietly in darkness, a cold compress, acetaminophen or ibuprofen, narcotic analgesics, sleep, massage, and even exercise have been reported to be helpful. Children with migraine seek a dark, quiet room, a cold compress, and sleep. Adolescents with chronic muscle contraction headaches may find little relief with medication. Some find sleep of temporary benefit.

(15) Does anything make the headaches worse?

Behaviors that exacerbate pain need to be identified. In many patients with headache, stress, bright lights, noise, and strenuous activity make the pain worse.

(16) Do symptoms continue between headaches?

Progressive headaches of an organic nature need to be differentiated from those that are paroxysmal or from those that are static and nonprogressive. Increased intracranial pressure or a mass lesion will have progressive symptoms, such as personality change, forgetfulness, lethargy, visual difficulty, nausea, balance difficulty, and weakness. The presence of neurologic symptoms or signs between the headaches is significant.

(17) Are you being treated for or do you have any other medical problems?

Allergy may be associated with headache secondary to sinusitis. Hypertension can cause intermittent or chronic headaches.

(18) Do you take medication for any other problem on a regular basis or on an intermittent basis?

Stimulants for ADD, bronchodilators for asthma, or illicit drugs can cause headache. Daily use of over-the-counter medication can cause or worsen some headaches. Nonsteroidal anti-inflammatory drugs (NSAIDs), antihypertensives, and antidepressants can cause headache.[12]

(19) Does anyone else in the family have headaches?

Migraine is often genetic. Chronic nonprogressive headaches occur in stressful environments. Do parents, siblings, grandparents, or other relatives have a history of headaches currently or earlier in their lives? The parents need to obtain information from relatives. It must be noted whether those headaches occurred on a daily basis or were "sick headaches" with nausea and vomiting (migraine).

(20) What do you think is causing your headaches?

Fears that the patient may have about a brain tumor need to be elicited. Intuitive children know that their headaches are due to self-imposed or externally imposed stress at school or in the family.

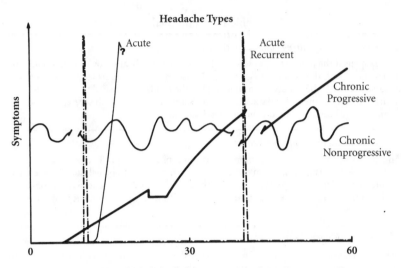

Figure 2–1   Types of headaches according to temporal patterns.

Increased Intracranial Pressure

Symptoms of increased intracranial pressure or progressive neurologic symptoms need to be determined.[13] Progressive lethargy, personality change, nausea, vomiting, visual difficulties, focal weakness, or ataxia are important. Any hint of symptoms of increased intracranial pressure or progressive neurologic disease strongly suggest the need for an in-depth evaluation including neuroimaging.

Family History

In addition to the data previously obtained regarding other family members with headache, a family history of hypertension, allergy, collagen vascular disease, epilepsy, tumor, and neurocutaneous disorders may be useful.

Medical History

Details concerning pregnancy, labor and delivery, growth and development, previous injuries (especially head injuries), operations, hospitalizations, serious illnesses, drug allergies or reactions, current medications, use of illicit drugs or alcohol, convulsions, or other neurologic problems should be obtained. A detailed review of organ systems is necessary to establish whether they are causing the headaches. For example, hypertension, sinus infections, chronic pulmonary problems, heart murmurs, eye infections, chronic ear infections, allergies, epilepsy, diabetes, or head trauma may be the source of the headaches.[14] A prior history of chronic limb pain or abdominal pain for which no cause was found may indicate stress.[15]

Other questions that need to be asked include the following: Is the child in an appropriate grade or special class? Is the patient getting straight As or failing? Has there been a change in the patient's school or schoolwork? How hard does the patient need to work to obtain good grades? Are there pressures to obtain high grades from internal or external sources? Does the patient leave school in the middle of the day? Has the patient missed an inordinate number of school days? Is the patient home schooled?

Emotional factors are critical. Does the child have close friends and interact with them regularly? If there has been a change in behavior or depression, drug abuse should be considered.[16] Truancy, divorce, abuse, recent deaths in the family, and peer suicide also may lead to headache. Symptoms of depression, which include sadness, tearfulness, withdrawal from activities, hopelessness and helplessness, need to be checked.[16]

The examiner should have tentatively classified the headache type at the conclusion of the history (see Figures 2–1 and 2–2).

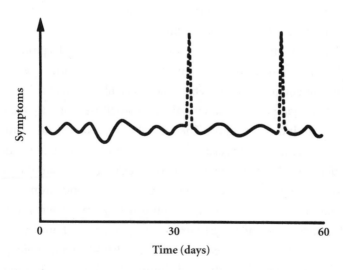

Figure 2–2   The mixed headache syndrome. Chronic nonprogressive.

PHYSICAL EXAMINATION

The examiners should keep in mind the tentative diagnosis and substantiate their clinical impression while performing the general examination.[17,18] Fever may indicate an infectious process. Elevated blood pressure can cause headaches. If the child's height and weight are significantly above or below the average, consider a pituitary or hypothalamic disorder. Conditions such as asthma and their medications may play a role in the pathogenesis of headache. Hyperventilation is indicative of anxiety. Petechia may indicate a blood dyscrasia with bleeding. Striae may indicate Cushing's disease or illicit use of steroids. Five or more café-au-lait spots may implicate neurofibromatosis; the presence of a butterfly rash, vasculitis; and organomegaly, a systemic neoplasm. In other words, headache may be a nonspecific symptom of disease in any organ system.

NEUROLOGIC EXAMINATION[19,20]

Observations regarding affect, response to questions, and ability to carry out commands are part of the mental status examination. Confusion, depression, and dementia can be identified prior to the formal neurologic examination.

Gait abnormalities can be seen in hemiparesis, ataxia, or hysteria. Posterior fossa lesions will cause a wide-based, unsteady gait. Difficulty arising from a knee bend indicates proximal weakness.

The head must be measured. If significantly enlarged, familial macrocephaly, compensated hydrocephalus, and neurofibromatosis are possibilities. The presence of an asymmetric machinery-like cranial bruit may indicate an underlying vascular abnormality. Localized areas of scalp tenderness or fluid may indicate trauma. The cranial nerve examination should be adjusted, depending on the age and cooperation of the patient. In young or uncooperative children, the funduscopic examination should be performed at the end of the neurologic examination. Optic atrophy, hemorrhage, diminished visual acuity, or abnormal eye movements indicate a need for further testing. If dysfunction or asymmetry is found at any level of the neuraxis—motor, sensory, or cerebellar—a pathologic process should be suspected. The pattern of abnormality allows localization.

In the majority of patients with tension or migraine headaches, the general physical and neurologic examinations are normal.

EMERGENCY EVALUATION[21–23]

Two to 6% of emergency department (ED) visits are due to headache. Emergency department headaches in the pediatric and adolescent population are due to non–central nervous system infections, central nervous system infections, trauma, acute vascular insults, shunt malfunction, increased intracranial pressure, tension, or migraine.

In the ED the headache history is directed toward ruling out organic disease and life-threatening illness. If the patient's sensorium is altered, the patient is in severe pain, or the clinical condition is precarious, the history is truncated. Is this the first or worst headache of the patient's life? Has it been associated with chronic sinusitis and now with a stiff neck and fever? Was it a "sudden thunderclap" headache now associated with a stiff neck and altered sensorium or is it an acute exacerbation of headaches that have been occurring for several years? The character of the headache, its severity, duration and associated symptoms should be outlined. Specific questions concerning illicit drugs, medications, and exertion should be obtained.

Fever, elevated blood pressure, and signs of trauma are noted. The neck should be carefully checked for stiffness. Pupillary responses and funduscopic examination are critical. The presence of generalized or focal neurologic signs indicates the presence of an underlying neurologic disease. The history and physical examination dictate the choice of diagnostic tests.

Critical conditions requiring emergency intervention include subarachnoid hemorrhage, meningitis, brain abscess, hypertension, hydrocephalus, and increased intracranial pressure.

At the conclusion of the history and examinations, a differential diagnosis should be formulated. Does the patient have a tension headache, migraine, or is an "organic" headache either secondary to a systemic disorder or an intracranial abnormality? Laboratory tests should be chosen to confirm a diagnosis or to rule out a potentially life-threatening disorder. Routine testing is rarely valuable in making the diagnosis or in convincing patients that they do not have an organic disorder.

LABORATORY TESTS[24]

The choice of laboratory tests rests on the differential diagnosis suggested by the history, the character and temporal pattern of the headache, and the physical and neurologic examinations. Routine blood work, including complete blood count, sequential multiple analysis of 17 constituents or a general metabolic profile, sedimentation rate, and antinuclear antibody profile, is not helpful in patients who have migraine or chronic nonprogressive headaches or no symptoms of increased pressure and normal examinations. If the patient is ill, these studies may be of value. Other blood tests useful in specific circumstances include serum lead, carbon monoxide, and toxicology screen.

The electroencephalogram (EEG) is of limited value in the routine evaluation of headaches.[25] Nonspecific abnormalities are frequently found in many normal children.[26] If the patient's headache disorder is associated with loss of consciousness, alteration of consciousness, and/or abnormal movements, the differential diagnosis may include seizures. An EEG may be useful, but it is important to recognize that up to 10% of patients with migraine may have benign focal epileptiform discharges that are not related to seizures or headache.[27] Evoked potentials and brain electrical activity mapping have not proven to be of clinical value and should not be routinely performed.[28,29]

NEUROIMAGING

The diagnosis of hydrocephalus or a mass lesion has been revolutionized with the development of computed tomography (CT) and magnetic resonance imaging (MRI). Skull roentgenograms, radioisotope scanning, positron emission tomography scanning, arteriography, pneumoencephalography, and digital subtraction angiography are rarely needed.

Computed tomography is a safe, rapid, accurate method of evaluating intracranial contents.[30,31] It is useful in a wide variety of disorders, including congenital malformations, cranial infections, trauma, neoplasms, and vascular disorders. In the acute situation where hemorrhage is suspected, it may be a lifesaving procedure. Magnetic resonance imaging is valuable when an imaging procedure is needed and time is not of the essence. Although it is more costly, takes longer, and may require sedation, it may demonstrate sellar lesions, craniocervical junction lesions, white matter abnormalities, and congenital anomalies more accurately than CT scanning.[32,33] Magnetic resonance imaging also demonstrates sinus pathology without extra cuts. The majority of patients who have migraine or those who have chronic nonprogressive headaches with no symptoms of progressive neurologic dysfunction, no symptoms of increased intracranial pressure, and a normal neurologic examination do not require imaging. Indeed, the overwhelming number of studies in these patients are normal or show unrelated abnormalities.[33]

In patients with histories suggestive of a vascular event, magnetic resonance arteriography should be done.[34] If pseudotumor cerebri or venous obstruction is suspected, magnetic resonance venography can be diagnostic.

Lumbar puncture is useful in determining the presence of infection, blood, or increased pressure.[35] If a space-occupying lesion is suspected, the lumbar puncture may be contraindicated and should be preceded by a neuroimaging procedure. In the event of an acute infectious process where bacterial meningitis is the primary diagnosis, the lumbar puncture should be performed without waiting for the scan. If pseudotumor cerebri is suspected, the pressure measurement is critical and reassurance or sedation may be needed.

Psychologic tests are useful in children and adolescents who have chronic nonprogressive headaches or are suspected of having headaches associated with known stressful circumstances.[36] When school problems coexist, psychoeducational testing is indicated. Personality tests such as the Minnesota Multiphasic Personality Inventory—Adolescent and the Parent Inventory for Children are used to identify or confirm stressors.

At the conclusion of the history, physical examination, and laboratory tests, the specific headache type should be confirmed and its etiology known or suspected (see Figures 2–1 and 2–2). Treatment can be initiated. It may be simple observation involving asking the patient to maintain a headache calendar, avoid specific foods, or use over-the-counter medication judiciously. A follow-up contact in 4 to 6 weeks is useful. If specific symptoms require treatment, they can be initiated. Both the child and the parent need to understand the timing, dosages, uses, and misuses of medications, their common side effects, and their potential serious side effects.

Patient/parent education and written instructions are valuable. If medication is prescribed, a follow-up contact is useful. At that time, the headache problem should be reviewed. If its character is changing or if new neurologic symptoms or signs have appeared, neuroimaging or other testing, if not previously done, can be considered. If the patients' headaches have been responsive to general measures, the patients can be followed by their primary care physician. If the patients are being treated with prophylactic migraine medication or antidepressants, a plan for monitoring and later discontinuation of those medications and follow-up should be discussed.

In the vast majority of children and adolescents, a thorough history and complete physical and neurologic examination will identify the headache type.

REFERENCES

1. Dodge PR. Neurologic history and examination. In: Farmer TW, ed. Pediatric Neurology. New York: Harper and Row, 1964, pp 3–64.
2. Lance JW. Recording the patient's case history. In: Mechanism and Management of Headache, 4th ed. Boston: Butterworth Scientific, 1982, pp 8–15.
3. Bana DS, Leviton A, Swidler C, et al. A computer-based headache interview: acceptance by patients and physicians. Headache 1980;20(2):85–89.
4. Schechter NL. Recurrent pains in children: an overview and approach. Pediatr Clin North Am 1984;31:949.
5. Richardson GM, McGrath PJ, Cunningham SJ, Humphreys P. Validity of the headache diary for children. Headache 1983;23:184–187.
6. Newman LC, Lipton RB, Solomon S. Headache history and neurological examination. In: Tollison CD, Kunkel RS, eds. Headache: Diagnosis and Treatment. Baltimore: Williams & Wilkins, 1993, pp 23–30.
7. Lance JW. Pattern recognition from the history. In: Mechanism and Management of Headache, 4th ed. Boston: Butterworth Scientific, 1982, pp 16–21.
8. Rothner AD. Headaches in children: a review. Headache 1979;19:156.
9. Hachinski VC, Porchawka J, Steele JC. Visual symptoms in the migraine syndrome. Neurology 1973;23:570.
10. Bieri D, Reeve RA, Champion GD, et al. The faces pain scale for the self-assessment of the severity of pain experienced by children: development, initial validation, and preliminary investigation for ratio scale properties. Pain 1990;41:139–150.

11. Mathews JR, McGrath PJ, Pigeon H. Assessment and measurement of pain in children. In: Schecter NL, Berde CB, Yaster M, eds. Pain in Infants, Children, and Adolescents. Baltimore: Williams & Wilkins, 1993, pp 97–111.

12. Mathew N, Kurman R, Perez F. Drug-induced refractory headache—clinical features and management. Headache 1990;30:634–638.

13. Rosman NP. Increased intracranial pressure in childhood. Pediatr Clin North Am 1974;21:483–499.

14. Solomon GD. Concomitant medical disease and headache. Med Clin North Am 1991;75:631–639.

15. Sherry DD, McGuire T, Mellins E. Psychosomatic musculoskeletal pain in childhood: clinical and psychological analyses of 100 children. Pediatrics 1991;88:1093–1099.

16. Ling W, Oftedal G, Weinberg W. Depressive illness in childhood presenting as severe headache. Am J Dis Child 1970;120:122–124.

17. Hockelman RA. The physical examination of infants and children. In: Bickley LS, Hoekelman RA, eds. Physical Examination and History Taking, 7th ed. New York: Lippincott, 1974, pp 621–704.

18. Barness LA. Manual of Pediatric Physical Diagnosis, 5th ed. Chicago: Year Book Medical, 1980.

19. Paine RS, Oppé TE. Neurological examination of children. Clin Dev Med 1966;20:21.

20. Swaiman KF. Neurologic examination of the older child. In: Swaimann KF, Ashwal S. Pediatric Neurology: Principles and Practice: 2, 3rd ed. St. Louis, MO: Mosby, 1999.

21. Rothner AD. Headache emergencies: evaluation, differential diagnosis, and treatment. In: Current Management in Child Neurology. London: B.C. Decker, 1999, pp 331–335.

22. Diamond ML. Emergency treatment of headache. In: The Practicing Physician's Approach to Headache, 5th ed. Baltimore: Williams & Wilkins, 1992, pp 259–269.

23. Dhopesh V, Anwar R, Herring C. A retrospective assessment of emergency department patients with complaint of headache. Headache 1979;19:37–42.

24. Menkes JH. Neurologic examination of the child and infant. In: Menkes JH, Sarnat HB, eds. Textbook of Child Neurology, 6th ed. Philadelphia: Williams & Wilkins, 1995, pp 1–32.

25. DeRomanis F, Buzzi MG, Assensa S, et al. Basilar migraine with electroencephalographic findings of occipital spike-wave complexes: a long-term study in seven children. Cephalalgia 1993;13:192–196.

26. Eeg-Oloffsson O. The development of the electroencephalogram in normal adolescents from the age of 16 through 21 years. Neuropadiatrie 1971;3:11.

27. Kinast M, Lueders H, Rothner AD, et al. Benign focal epileptiform discharges in childhood migraine (BFEDC). Neurology 1982;32:1309.

28. Battistella PA, Suppiej A, Gianluca C, et al. Brainstem auditory evoked potentials (BAEPs) in childhood migraine. Headache 1988;28:204–206.

29. Binnie CD, Macgillivray BB. Brain mapping—a useful tool or a dangerous toy? J Neurol Neurosurg Psychiatr 1992;55:527–529.

30. Dooley JM, Camfield PR, O'Neill M, Vohra A. The value of CT scans for children with headaches. Can J Neurol Sci 1990;17:309–310.

31. Weingarten S, Kleinman M, Elperin L, Larson EB. The effectiveness of cerebral imaging in the diagnosis of chronic headache. Arch Intern Med 1992;152:2457–2462.

32. Osborn RE, Alder DC, Mitchell CS. MR imaging of the brain in patients with migraine headaches. AJNR Am J Neuroradiol 1991;12:521–524.

33. Practice parameter: the utility of neuroimaging in the evaluation of headache in patients with normal neurologic examinations (summary statement). Report of the Quality Standards Subcommittee of the American Academy of Neurology. Neurology 1994;44:1353–1354.

34. Ruggieri PM, Masaryk TJ, Ross JS, Modic MT. Intracranial magnetic resonance angiography. Cardiovasc Intervent Radiol 1992;15:71–81.

35. Portnoy JM, Olson LC. Normal cerebrospinal fluid values in children: another look. Pediatrics 1985;75:484.

36. Harrison RH. Psychological testing in headache: a review. Headache 1975;14:177.

Chapter 3

SECONDARY HEADACHES

A. David Rothner
and Andrew Hershey

Secondary headaches are also called "organic headaches."[1] These headaches, unlike many of the others discussed in this book, have an etiology that can often be identified. The International Headache Society (IHS) differentiated them from the primary headache types of migraine, tension, and cluster.[2] These headaches can be grouped in three different ways: etiology, symptom complex, and temporal presentation.[1,3,4] In this chapter, we review secondary headaches and identify their unique characteristics.

The medical model for the evaluation of headaches includes a thorough history. In the case of secondary headaches, special attention must be given to symptoms of increased intracranial pressure and progressive neurologic dysfunction. If the headache is of recent onset and increasing in severity or frequency, awakens the patient at night, always occurs in the morning, is associated with projectile vomiting, is described by the patient as the "worst headache ever," or is associated with straining, then an organic disorder should be suspected.[1,4] During the physical examination, in addition to a thorough general pediatric examination and neurologic examination, special attention should be paid to evidence of trauma and meningismus. The differential diagnosis depends on the clinical presentation. These secondary headaches may present acutely, subacutely, or in a chronic progressive fashion. Table 3–1 lists the categories of secondary headaches as outlined by the IHS.[2] Table 3–2 is a mnemonic that many practitioners find useful in separating secondary headaches into subcategories. Table 3–3 arranges these categories by temporal presentation.[4]

The neurologic history and examination leads to the differential diagnosis that indicates which diagnostic tests should be performed.

Table 3–1   Secondary Headaches

Trauma
Vascular disorders
Hydrocephalus
Intracranial infection
Neoplasm
Substance use
Metabolic disorder
Hypoxia
Disorders of cranium (e.g., sinuses, eyes, etc.)

Adapted from: Classification and diagnostic criteria for headache disorders, cranial neuralgias and facial pain. Headache Classification Committee of the International Headache Society. Cephalalgia 1988;8(Suppl 7):9–96.

OFFICE SETTING

The primary care physician in the office setting has the responsibility of differentiating organic headaches secondary to commonly encountered, non–life-threatening disorders from those that are more serious. Headaches in the office setting are quite common and most are not due to "serious" problems.[3,5–7] Frequent or severe headache follows allergy, otitis media, asthma, and eczema in order or prevalence. This can cause a significant number of missed school days. Of interest is the fact that the majority of children with mild to moderate headache do not seek medical care. Psychosocial stress plays an important role. The majority of headaches

Table 3–2   Secondary Headaches by Category

C	Congenital anomalies (e.g., hydrocephalus, Arnold-Chiari)
I	Infection (e.g., meningitis, abscess)
T	Toxin (e.g., cocaine, amphetamines)
T	Trauma (e.g., subdural, epidural)
E	Endocrine (e.g., hypoglycemia)
N	Neoplasm (e.g., brain tumor, leukemia)
D	Degenerative disorder (e.g., Alexander's disease)
V	Vascular (e.g., aneurysm, arteriovenous malformation, coagulation disorder)
M	Metabolic (e.g., hypoxia, dehydration, fever)

Table 3–3   Acute Headache

A Acute Generalized	B Acute Localized
Systemic infection	Sinusitis
Central nervous system infection	Otitis
Toxins (e.g., lead, CO)	Ocular abnormality
Postseizure	Dental disease
Electrolyte imbalance	Trauma
Hypertension	Occipital neuralgia
Hypoglycemia	Temporomandibular
Postlumbar puncture	joint disorder
Trauma	
Embolism	
Vascular thrombosis	
Hemorrhage	
Collagen disease	
Exertion	
Shunt malfunction	
C Recurrent	D Chronic Progressive
Vascular disease	Tumor
Intoxication	Pseudotumor
MELAS	Brain abscess
Postseizure	Subdural hematoma
Hypoglycemia	Hydrocephalus
Exertion	

CO = carbon monoxide; MELAS = mitochondrial encephalopathy, lactic acidosis, and stroke-like attacks.

seen in the primary care physician's office without symptoms of increased intracranial pressure or progressive neurologic disease can be managed without difficulty. In a study of 37 children, Kandt and Levine indicated that 30% of children coming to the primary care physician's office with headache had non–central nervous system infection.[5] Infectious disorders were important in 22 of 37 patients and included viral infections, pharyngitis, otitis, and sinusitis. Patients with family histories of migraine were more likely to have headache. Sleep disorders were more common in headache patients than nonheadache patients. Because headache is often seen in the primary care physician's office, further studies of this nature are needed. Mild trauma without neurologic symptoms or signs is also common, as are headaches secondary to medications and substance abuse. It should be emphasized that ocular disease and serious medical and/or neurologic problems are indeed uncommon in the otherwise well child presenting to the primary care physician's office. To properly evaluate the child requires assessment of school performance and psychologic factors, as well as medical factors.

EMERGENCY DEPARTMENT

Four studies have been published looking at the frequency, etiology, and evaluation of headaches in children and adolescents presenting to the emergency department.[8–11] Once again, these children may have the acute onset of headache, an acute recurrent presentation, or a chronic progressive presentation. The differential diagnosis of each of these categories is seen in Table 3–3 under subheadings A, B, C, and D. Approximately 5% of all children presenting to the emergency department have the chief complaint of headache. Of this group, anywhere from 2 to 15% have serious underlying medical and/or neurologic problems as the etiology of their headaches. The remainder have a variety of conditions including stress-related headaches, migraine, headaches associated with infectious disorders, and mild trauma. The etiologies of significant neurologic or medical conditions include hydrocephalus, shunt malfunction, aseptic meningitis, bacterial meningitis, brain abscess, substance abuse, trauma, metabolic dysfunction, neoplasms, and vascular disorders.

The following conditions should be included in the differential diagnosis of secondary headaches.

Congenital Malformations

Several nonvascular congenital malformations may result in either acute headache or chronic progressive headache. Prominent among them are hydrocephalus and the Arnold-Chiari malformation. Hydrocephalus is a ventricular dilation caused by obstruction of cerebrospinal fluid (CSF) flow or its absorption.[12] With this syndrome, there is a progressive increase in intracranial pressure, which results in headache, nausea, vomiting, lethargy, ataxia, and macrocephaly. It may present acutely or be variably progressive.

In younger children, the usual presentation involves a rapidly enlarging head circumference, vomiting, lethargy, and irritability. The latter is an expression of headache in the younger child. In older children and adolescents, headache, lethargy, vomiting, and diplopia may be present. On neurologic examination, macrocephaly, papilledema, and sixth nerve palsies may be present. If this diagnosis is suspected, an imaging procedure is necessary. Treatment of this condition requires a CSF diversion procedure, such as a shunt or a third ventriculostomy.

Children or adolescents who have already been shunted for hydrocephalus and present with headache, either in the primary physician's office or emergency department, are a diagnostic dilemma.[13,14] Does the patient have an infectious process, stress-related headaches, migraine, or shunt malfunction? Although this problem has been addressed in several articles in the literature, the diagnostic approach is difficult. The patient should be considered to have shunt malfunction until an alternate etiology is identified.

The Arnold-Chiari malformation is being identified with increasing frequency with the increased use of magnetic resonance imaging (MRI).[15] Not all patients with the Arnold-Chiari malformation have headaches secondary to their deformity. Diligence is required to establish that headaches in a child are secondary to the Arnold-Chiari malformation. Common symptoms include headache in the occipital region and the neck, upper extremity weakness, gait disturbance, and at times, sensory complaints. Symptoms may also be referable to the spinal cord, and an associated syringomyelia may be present. Although the headache may be chronic and aggravated by straining, such as from coughing, running, or hyperextension of the neck, these symptoms are not diagnostic. Magnetic resonance imaging with CSF flow studies may be useful. Suboccipital decompression is necessary if the headaches are secondary to the malformation.

Infectious Disorders

Infectious disorders are commonly associated with headache. The presence of an elevated temperature and tachycardia frequently gives rise to a pounding headache, which is often relieved when the infection is treated and the temperature returns to normal.

Sinusitis

Acute sinusitis often presents with fever, rhinorrhea, and tenderness over the facial area, as well as headaches.[16] Children with this disorder often have a previous history of allergies and/or sinusitis. Maxillary sinusitis is the most common and is facial and frontal in location. Frontal sinusitis, which occurs in adolescents but not in children, includes pain in the forehead and top of the head. Sphenoid sinusitis pain occurs in the occipital region and vertex. In 1988, Faleck et al. reported on a review of 150 children and adolescents with chronic headache.[17] Sinus pathology was present in 10% of patients, all of whom improved with antibiotic therapy. Sinusitis should be considered in the differential diagnosis of children and adolescents with chronic headache.

Meningitis

With the availability of newer vaccines, the incidence of bacterial meningitis has decreased.[18] It is not a common cause of headache in children or adolescents coming to the emergency department. Infants with meningitis will often present with fever, lethargy, irritability, and a bulging fontanel. Neck stiffness may be present. The older child or adolescent with bacterial meningitis presents with a severe headache that increases rapidly. It is usually generalized and associated with pain in the neck. On examination, these patients may have nuchal rigidity and a positive Kernig's sign and Brudzinski's sign. If the diagnosis of bacterial meningitis is suspected and there is no consideration of a mass lesion, lumbar puncture should be done as soon as possible. This diagnosis should be suspected, especially in individuals who have skull fractures or chronic sinusitis or who are immunocompromised.

Aseptic Meningitis and Encephalitis[19,20]

These disorders usually present with headache, fever, and stiff neck. In aseptic meningitis, mental status changes are not usually present. In encephalitis, seizures, mental status changes, and focal neurologic signs are prominent. Headaches are common in both of these disorders and may be the initial presenting symptom. These disorders must be recognized quickly because, in the case of herpes encephalitis, delay in diagnosis may lead to severe neurologic sequelae. In the latter, electroencephalography is helpful, and specific therapy is available.

Many of these disorders have a seasonal presentation or relate to childhood exanthems. Once suspected, in the majority of instances, the diagnosis can be confirmed by lumbar puncture demonstrating abnormal CSF. It should be emphasized that Lyme disease, cat-scratch disease, and rickettsial disease may affect the central nervous system and present with severe headache, meningismus, and abnormal CSF. These disorders may be difficult to distinguish from viral meningitis and may present without a history of tick exposure or rash.[21]

Brain Abscess

Brain abscess may present acutely or subacutely.[22] It occurs more commonly in children or adolescents with cyanotic congenital heart disease, penetrating head trauma, chronic ear infections, chronic pulmonary disease, postneurosurgical procedures, or in children who are immunocompromised. Headache and generalized or focal neurologic symptoms and signs are usual. If a brain abscess is suspected, an MRI scan with and without gadolinium enhancement should be performed and a lumbar puncture avoided because of the risk of herniation. Management involves antibiotics and surgical drainage, as well as the concomitant treatment of any associated seizure disorders.

Substance-Induced Headache

Medication and illicit drugs an cause headache.[23,24] These may be medications used to treat illnesses and/or substances that are being abused. The IHS groups medication-induced headaches under the title of "Headache Associated with Substances or Their Withdrawal." Medication may initiate a headache, exacerbate a pre-existing headache, or cause a headache on its withdrawal. This subject was reviewed by Silberstein in 1998.[23] Of interest is that medications used to treat headache, such as indomethacin, caffeine, corticosteroids, selective serotonin reuptake inhibitors, antibiotics, and β-blockers, can themselves cause headache.

Chronic drug-induced headache may occur with overuse of symptomatic medications, as defined by the regular daily intake of simple analgesics or combination analgesics containing barbiturates or sedatives more than four times weekly. Medications implicated include barbiturates, narcotics, ergotamine, and even acetaminophen, salicylates, and nonsteroidal anti-inflammatory drugs. These medications can cause headaches when they are used on a regular basis or when suddenly stopped. Chronic drug-induced headache has been reported less often in children and adolescents. Special attention should be directed to medication-related idiopathic intracranial hypertension (pseudotumor cerebri). Steroids, hormones, outdated antibiotics, and vitamins have all been causally related.

Headaches are seen in the patient with substance abuse with or without associated neurologic symptoms. Cocaine, heroin, and amphetamines are most commonly implicated.

Trauma

Trauma is a common occurrence in infants, children, and adolescents. It may occur accidentally during sports or play or be secondary to child abuse.[25] The headaches may occur immediately after or within months of the head injury. Post-traumatic headaches are reviewed in Chapter 9. Headaches occurring soon after trauma frequently involve loss of consciousness, post-traumatic amnesia, or abnormal neurologic symptoms and signs.

Acute post-traumatic headache after minor head trauma is characterized by vomiting, headache, and malaise. The symptoms in the absence of serious underlying neurologic problems usually resolve quickly. It should be noted that in the genetically predisposed, head trauma may initiate migraine or precipitate migraine in a patient already known to have migraine.[26] If serious head trauma has occurred, cortical contusions and subdural and epidural hematomas enter into the differential diagnosis. The presentation is usually acute and associated with neurologic symptoms and signs.

Neoplasms

Intracranial tumors are the second most common type of neoplasm in children.[27,28] In children younger than 15 years, the incidence is 2.4 per 100,000. Certain genetic syndromes, such as neurofibromatosis, tuberous sclerosis, von Hippel-Lindau disease, and ataxia telangiectasia pose a greater risk for the development of neoplasms.

The fear of brain tumor is a major concern of parents bringing their children to the pediatrician for evaluation of headache.[29] Although a clear association between brain tumors and headaches exists, the overwhelming majority of headaches are not caused by tumors. When a brain tumor causes a headache, it is usually secondary to increased intracranial pressure due to the mass itself or secondary to obstruction of CSF flow.[1] The rapidity with which this takes place affects the temporal presentation of the patient. The headache pattern is usually chronic and progressive and increases in frequency and severity over time. It may be present at any time in the day but is frequently reported to occur in the morning. Mild analgesics may provide relief early in the course of this disorder. Other symptoms include seizures, ataxia, weakness, visual abnormalities, lethargy, and personality change. In the majority of patients, the neurologic examination will be abnormal, and the diagnosis can be confirmed by neuroimaging. Non-neoplastic mass lesions may present in a similar fashion.

Vascular Disorders

Vascular disorders are frequently associated with headache.[30] The frequency of cerebrovascular diseases in children is 2.5 cases per 100,000. Disorders in this category include vasculitis, hypertension, thrombosis, emboli, and hemorrhage, the latter being secondary to aneurysms, vascular malformations, and trauma.

Vasculitis is uncommon in children and adolescents and usually occurs in the setting of an autoimmune disorder such as systemic lupus erythematosus, polyarteritis, Wegener's granulomatosis, and Sjögren's syndrome.[31] Although headaches may be the initial symptom, other systemic symptoms and signs are usually present. The headaches may resemble either chronic tension headaches or migraine and usually exacerbate when the underlying autoimmune disorder worsens. Headaches occur in 40 to 70% of patients with vasculitis. Other neurologic symptoms may include behavioral disorders, seizures, and focal deficits. Cerebrospinal fluid may be abnormal and angiography may show abnormalities. Corticosteroids and immunosuppressive agents are required.

Systemic hypertension, either acute or chronic, may be associated with headaches.[32] This is not common in the pediatric/adolescent population in the absence of underlying renal disease. Efforts should be addressed to identify the primary disorder. In the malignant hypertension syndrome, severe headache and lethargy are associated with papilledema, as well as retinal changes and hematuria. The differential diagnosis includes renal disease, coarctation of the aorta, pheochromocytoma, and cocaine or amphetamine abuse.

Thrombosis and emboli can be idiopathic or occur in relation to trauma, coagulation disorders, autoimmune disorders, and congenital heart disease.[33] Conditions such as moyamoya disease, fibromuscular dysplasia, tumor, trauma, sickle cell anemia, hemophilia, and dehydration may also be contributory. Migraine, especially in occurrence with other risk factors (e.g., hyperlipidemia, smoking, birth control pills), can be associated with stroke.

Hemorrhage may be secondary to rupture of a vascular malformation or aneurysm or secondary to trauma.[34] The presenting symptom is a severe headache often associated with loss of consciousness, meningismus, and focal neurologic symptoms. An underlying neurocutaneous disorder should be sought. If this diagnosis is suspected, a computed tomography scan will usually show the intracranial hemorrhage. Magnetic resonance imaging, magnetic resonance angiography, magnetic resonance venography (MRV), and angiography may delineate the specific etiology.

Venous sinus thrombosis may occur in the presence of an underlying metabolic or systemic infection or a coagulation disorder or as a result of dehydration.[33] The patients usually present with headaches, alteration of consciousness, focal neurologic symptoms, and seizures. The neurologic examination is usually abnormal and MRI, as well as MRV, will often show the thrombosed vessel. Consideration should be given to this diagnosis in the presence of a coagulopathy or chemotherapy.

Subdural, epidural, or intra-axial hematomas usually result from head trauma but may also occur secondary to rupture of a vascular malformation or aneurysm or in children with blood dyscrasia.[35,36] The usual symptoms include those of increased intracranial pressure; the abnormal signs include papilledema, retinal hemorrhages, focal neurologic abnormalities, and alteration of consciousness.

Pseudotumor Cerebri

Pseudotumor cerebri is also known as "benign intracranial hypertension." The headaches may be intermittent or constant and are often progressive.[37,38] Visual obscurations and tinnitus may occur. On examination, most patients have papilledema, changes in their visual fields, and a sixth nerve palsy. This disorder has been reported without papilledema.[38] Magnetic resonance imaging and MRV should be performed. A lumbar puncture should also be done. The goal of treatment is to preserve vision, decrease the intracranial pressure, and alleviate the headache. These patients require multiple treatment modalities, including lumbar punctures, weight loss, corticosteroids, and diuretics. If vision is deteriorating, a lumbar peritoneal shunt or optic nerve sheath decompression may be needed.

It should be noted that headaches secondary to decreased CSF pressure, as seen in spontaneous subarachnoid leaks or after lumbar puncture, are not uncommon in children and adolescents.[39] The patient's headache often worsens when he or she sits up, stands up, or exercises and is often relieved when the patient returns to the recumbent position. The headache can often be treated with analgesics and bed rest with spontaneous closure of the tear. If, however, this treatment is unsuccessful, a blood patch may be necessary. The incidence of postlumbar puncture headaches can be reduced by using specialized smaller needles.

CONCLUSION

The majority of headaches in children and adolescents are not due to serious underlying medical or neurologic conditions. A thorough history and physical examination, coupled with appropriate laboratory tests, can often ensure that an organic or secondary headache is not the cause of the patient's problem.

REFERENCES

1. Cohen BH. Headaches as a symptom of neurological disease. Semin Pediatr Neurol 1995;2:144–150.

2. Classification and diagnostic criteria for headache disorders, cranial neuralgias and facial pain. Headache Classification Committee of the International Headache Society. Cephalalgia 1988;8(Suppl 7):9–96.

3. Gladstein J, Holden EW, Peralta L, Raven M. Diagnoses and symptom patterns in children presenting to a pediatric headache clinic. Headache 1993;33:497–500.

4. Rothner AD. The evaluation of headaches in children and adolescents. Semin Pediatr Neurol 1995;2:109–118.

5. Kandt R, Levine R. Headache and acute illness in children. J Child Neurol 1987;2:22–27.

6. Mortimer J, Jay J, Jaron A. Epidemiology of headache and childhood migraine in an urban general practice using Ad Hoc, Vahlquist and IHS criteria. Dev Med Child Neurol 1992;34:1095–1101.

7. Smith MS. Headaches. Pediatr Ann 1995;24:446–491.

8. Burton LJ, Quinn B, Pratt-Cheney JL, Pourani M. Headache etiology in a pediatric emergency department. Pediatr Emerg Care 1997;13:1–4.

9. Lewis DW, Qureshi F. Acute headache in children and adolescents presenting to the emergency department. Headache 2000;40:200–203.

10. Kan L, Nagelberg J, Maytal J. Headaches in a pediatric emergency department: etiology, imaging, and treatment. Headache 2000;40:25–29.

11. Clinical policy for the initial approach to adolescents and adults presenting to the emergency department with a chief complaint of headache. American College of Emergency Physicians. Ann Emerg Med 1996;27:821–844.

12. Milhorat TH. Hydrocephalus in pediatric neurology. Philadelphia: FA Davis, 1978, pp 99–135.

13. Abbott R, Epstein FJ, Wisoff JK. Chronic headaches associated with a functioning shunt: usefulness of pressure monitoring. Neurosurgery 1991;28:72.

14. Nowak TP, James HE. Migraine headaches in hydrocephalic children: a diagnostic dilemma. Childs Nerv Syst 1989;5:310–314.

15. Pascual J, Oterino A, Berciano J. Headache in type I Chiari malformation. Neurology 1992;42:1519–1521.

16. Wald ER, Milmore GJ, Bowen AD, et al. Acute maxillary sinusitis in children. N Engl J Med 1981;304:749–754.

17. Faleck H, Rothner AD, Erenberg G, et al. Headache and subacute sinusitis in children and adolescents. Headache 1988;28:96–98.

18. Adams WG, Daver KA, Cochi SL, et al. Decline of childhood *Haemophilus influenzae* type B (Hib) disease in the Hib vaccine era. JAMA 1993;269: 221–226.

19. Bale JR Jr. Viral infections of the nervous system. In: Swaiman KF, Ashwal S, eds. Pediatric Neurology: Principles & Practice: 2, 6th ed. St. Louis, MO: Mosby, 1999, pp 1001–1024.

20. Kennedy PG. A retrospective analysis of forty-six cases of herpes encephalitis seen in Glasgow between 1962 and 1985. QJM 1998;68:533–540.

21. Bleman AL, Iyer M, Coyle PK, et al. Neurologic manifestations in children with North American Lyme disease. Neurology 1993;43:2609–2614.

22. Takkok IH, Erbengi A. Management of brain abscess in children: review of 130 cases over a period of 21 years. Childs Nerv Syst 1992;8:411–416.

23. Silberstein SD. Drug-induced headache. Neurol Clin 1998;16:107–123.

24. Asmark H, Lundberg PO, Olsson S. Drug-related headache. Headache 1989; 29:441–444.

25. Lanser JBK, Jennekens-Schinkel A, Peters ACB. Headache after closed head injury in children. Headache 1998;28:176–179.

26. Haas DC, Pineda GS, Lourie H. Juvenile head trauma syndromes and their relationship to migraine. Arch Neurol 1975;32:727–730.

27. Honig PJ, Charney EB. Children with brain tumor headaches. Distinguishing features. Am J Dis Child 1982;136:121.

28. The epidemiology of headache among children with brain tumor. Headache in children with brain tumors. The Childhood Brain Tumor Consortium. J Neurooncol 1991;10:31–46.

29. Lewis DW, Middlebrook MT, Mehallick L, et al. Pediatric headaches: what do the children want? Headache 1996;36:224–230.

30. Roach ES, Riela AR. Pediatric Cerebrovascular Disorders. Armonk, NY: Futura Publishing, 1995.

31. Vazquez-Cruz J, Traboulssi H, De la Serna R, et al. A prospective study of chronic or recurrent headaches in systemic lupus erythematosus. Headache 1990;30:232–235.

32. Uhari M, Saukkonen AL, Koskimies O. Central nervous system involvement in severe arterial hypertension of childhood. Eur J Pediatr 1979;132:141–146.

33. Barron TP, Gusnard DA, Zimmerman RA, et al. Cerebral venous thrombosis in neonates and children. Pediatr Neurol 1992;8:112.

34. Roach ES, Riela AR. Intracranial hemorrhage. In: Roach ES, Riela AR, eds. Pediatric Cerebrovascular Disorders. Armonk, NY: Futura Publishing, 1995, pp 69–83.

35. Meyer FB, Sundt TM, Fode NC, et al. Cerebral aneurysms in childhood and adolescence. J Neurosurg 1989;70:420–425.

36. Dhellemmes P, Lejeune J-P, Christiaens J-L, et al. Traumatic extradural hematomas in infancy and childhood. J Neurosurg 1985;62:861–864.

37. Corbett JJ. Problems in the diagnosis and treatment of pseudotumor cerebri. Can J Neurol Sci 1983;10:221–229.
38. Marcelis J, Siberstein SD. Idiopathic intracranial hypertension without papilledema. Arch Neurol 1991;48:392–399.
39. Cassady JF, Lederhaas G, Turk WR, Shanks DE. Unusual presentation and treatment of postlumbar puncture headache in an 11-yr-old boy. Anesthesiology 2000;92:1835–1837.

Chapter 4

MIGRAINE PATHOPHYSIOLOGY

Peter J. Goadsby

K nowledge of migraine has expanded explosively in the last century.[1]
Therefore it is a key requirement to update physicians on the pathophysiology of migraine since understanding the disease can impact diagnosis and management.[2] Time is well spent understanding the mechanisms of headache given how common headache problems are and the
expansion of migraine treatments in the last few years.[3] The need for
understanding the disease is most striking in children and adolescents
because the clinical manifestations are more subtle and the recognition of
migraine requires a more searching clinical approach. Generally, the clinical features of migraine are less well developed in childhood: they are
sometimes characterized by shorter attacks or by less-associated features.
Although manageable, they are still a life-disabling, biologically determined condition.

The essential elements to be considered (Table 4–1) in understanding migraine are:

• anatomy of head pain, the large intracranial vessels, the dura mater, and
their trigeminovascular innervation;

• physiology and pharmacology of activation of the peripheral branches of
the ophthalmic branch of the trigeminal nerve as marked by plasma protein extravasation and neuropeptide release;

• physiology and pharmacology of the trigeminal nucleus, in particular
its caudal-most part, the trigeminocervical complex;

• central nervous system activation in association with pain in the thalamus and cortical areas; and

• brain stem and diencephalic modulatory systems that control trigeminal pain processing.

Table 4–1   Neuroanatomic Processing of Vascular Head Pain

Target Innervation	Structure	Comments
Cranial vessels and dura mater	Ophthalmic branch of trigeminal nerve	
1st	Trigeminal ganglion	Middle cranial fossa
2nd	Trigeminal nucleus (quintothalamic tract)	Trigeminal nucleus caudalis and C_1/C_2 dorsal horns
3rd	Thalamus	Ventrobasal complex, medial nucleus of posterior group, intralaminar complex
4th	Cortex	Insulae, frontal cortex, anterior cingulate cortex, basal ganglia

TRIGEMINOVASCULAR ANATOMY: STRUCTURES THAT PRODUCE PAIN

Surrounding the large cerebral vessels, pial vessels, large venous sinuses, and dura mater is a plexus of largely unmyelinated fibers that arise from the ophthalmic division of the trigeminal ganglion[4] and in the posterior fossa from the upper cervical dorsal roots.[5] Trigeminal fibers innervating cerebral vessels arise from neurons in the trigeminal ganglion that contain substance P and calcitonin gene-related peptide (CGRP),[6] both of which can be released when the trigeminal ganglion is stimulated either in humans or cats.[7] Stimulation of the cranial vessels, such as the superior sagittal sinus (SSS), is certainly painful in humans.[8] Human dural nerves that innervate the cranial vessels largely consist of small diameter myelinated and unmyelinated fibers that almost certainly subserve a nociceptive function.

What then is the source of pain in migraine? It must also be borne in mind that the pain process is likely to be a combination of direct factors, such as the activation of the nociceptors of pain-producing intracranial structures, in concert with a reduction in the normal functioning of the endogenous pain-control pathways that normally gate that pain.[9] Certainly, if the carotid artery is occluded ipsilateral to the side of headache in migraineurs, then two-thirds will experience relief, although this does not account for the other one-third.[10] Moreover, distension of major cerebral vessels by balloon dilatation leads to pain referred to the ophthalmic division of the trigeminal nerve.[11–13] There is little doubt that sufficient changes in vascular diameter would produce pain, but are the changes in migraine sufficient of themselves? The answer to the problem of pain generation is to be found in the physiology and pathophysiology of headache.

TRIGEMINOVASCULAR PHYSIOLOGY: PERIPHERAL CONNECTIONS

There is considerable experimental animal and human work that explains the physiology of activating trigeminal nociceptive afferents, allowing us to build a picture of what may happen during migraine.

Plasma Protein Extravasation

Moskowitz[14] has provided an elegant series of experiments to suggest that some component of the pain of migraine may be a form of sterile neurogenic inflammation. Neurogenic plasma extravasation can be seen during electrical stimulation of the trigeminal ganglion in the rat.[15] Plasma extravasation can be blocked by ergot alkaloids,[16] indomethacin,[17] acetylsalicylic acid,[17] and the serotonin (5-hydroxytryptamine)-1–like agonist, sumatriptan.[18] The pharmacology of the new abortive antimigraine drugs has been recently reviewed in detail.[19] In addition, there are structural changes in the dura mater that are seen with trigeminal ganglion stimulation, and these include mast cell degranulation[20] and changes in postcapillary venules, including platelet aggregation.[21] Although it is generally accepted that such changes, particularly the initiation of a sterile inflammatory response, would cause pain,[22,23] it is not clear whether this is sufficient of itself or if it requires other stimulators or promoters. In a recent report no changes are seen with retinal angiography during acute attacks of migraine or cluster headache,[24] although plasma extravasation in the retina, blockable by sumatriptan, could be seen after trigeminal ganglion stimulation in the rat. Clearly, blockade of neurogenic plasma protein extravasation is not completely predictive of antimigraine efficacy in humans as evidenced by the failure in clinical trials of substance P, neurokinin-1 antagonists,[25–28] specific protein plasma extravasation blockers, CP122,288[29] and 4991w93,[30] an endothelin antagonist,[31] and a neurosteroid ganaxolone.[32]

Neuropeptide Studies

Electrical stimulation of the trigeminal ganglion in both the human and cat leads to increases in extracerebral blood flow and local release of both CGRP and substance P (SP).[7] In the cat, trigeminal ganglion stimulation also increases cerebral blood flow[33] by a pathway traversing the greater superficial petrosal branch of the facial nerve again releasing a powerful vasodilator peptide, vasoactive intestinal polypeptide (VIP).[34] Interestingly, the VIP-ergic innervation of the cerebral vessels is predominantly anterior rather than posterior, and this may contribute to this region's vulnerability to spreading depression and, in part, explain why the aura is very often seen to commence posteriorly. Stimulation of the more specifically vascular pain-producing SSS increases cerebral blood flow and jugular vein CGRP levels.[35] Human evidence that CGRP is elevated in the headache phase of migraine,[36,37] cluster headache,[38,39] and chronic paroxysmal hemicrania[40] supports the view that the trigeminovascular system may be activated in a protective role in these conditions. It is of interest, in this regard, that compounds that have not shown activity in human migraine, notably the conformationally restricted analogue of sumatriptan, CP122,288,[41] and zolmitriptan, 4991w93,[42] were both ineffective inhibitors of CGRP release after SSS stimulation in the cat. Current indications are that the CGRP antagonist BIBN4096, a potent selective nonpeptide antagonist, may answer the question of whether blockade of CGRP receptors can abort acute migraine. This is an exciting prospect as it would usher in an age of acute medications that are nonvasoconstrictor.

TRIGEMINOVASCULAR PHYSIOLOGY: CENTRAL CONNECTIONS

The Trigeminocervical Complex

The sites within the brain stem that are responsible for craniovascular pain have been mapped in experimental animals, including the monkey, using Fos immunohistochemistry, a method for looking at activated cells. After meningeal irritation with blood, Fos expression is reported in the trigeminal nucleus caudalis;[43] however, after stimulation of the SSS, Fos-like immunoreactivity is seen in the trigeminal nucleus caudalis and in the dorsal horn at the C_1 and C_2 levels in the cat[44] and monkey.[45] These latter findings are in accord with similar data using 2-deoxy-D-glucose measurements with SSS stimulation.[46] They contribute to our view of the trigeminal nucleus extending beyond the traditional nucleus caudalis to the dorsal horn of the high cervical region in a functional continuum that includes a cervical extension that could be regarded as a trigeminal nucleus cervicalis. To complete the anatomic loop, we have seen that stimulation of a branch of C_2, the greater occipital nerve, increases metabolic activity in the same regions, that is the trigeminal nucleus caudalis and C_1 and C_2 dorsal horn, as is seen with SSS stimulation.[47] Thus, the same group of cells has input from both supratentorial, clearly trigeminally innervated structures, and from branches of the nerve roots of the high cervical spinal cord. This accounts for the referral of pain to the neck that is seen so commonly in the clinic. Moreover, stimulation of a lateralized structure, the middle meningeal artery, produces Fos expression bilaterally in both the cat and monkey brain,[48] a finding that is consistent with the fact that up to one-third of patients complain of bilateral pain. The group of cells could be regarded functionally as the trigeminocervical complex.

These data demonstrate that a substantial portion of the trigemino-vascular nociceptive information comes by way of the most caudal cells. This concept provides an anatomic explanation for the referral of pain to the back of the head in migraine. Moreover, experimental pharmacologic evidence suggests that some abortive antimigraine drugs, such as ergots,[49] acetylsalicylic acid,[50] sumatriptan after blood-brain barrier disruption,[51] eletriptan,[52] naratriptan,[53,54] rizatriptan,[55] and zolmitriptan,[56] can have actions at these second-order neurons that reduce cell activity, suggesting also a further possible site for therapeutic intervention in migraine.

Thalamus

Following transmission in the caudal brain stem and high cervical spinal cord, information is relayed in a group of fibers (the quintothalamic tract) to the thalamus. Processing of vascular pain in the thalamus occurs in the ventroposteromedial thalamus, medial nucleus of the posterior complex, and the intralaminar thalamus.[57] Zagami and Lambert[58] have shown by application of capsaicin to the SSS that trigeminal projections with a high degree of nociceptive input are processed in neurons, particularly in the ventroposteromedial thalamus and its ventral periphery. Human imaging studies have confirmed activation of the thalamus contralateral to pain in acute cluster headache[59] and in SUNCT (short-lasting unilateral neuralgiform headache with conjunctival injection and tearing).[60]

Cortex

Pain, in general, is a complex phenomenon that is mediated by a network of neuronal structures, including the cingulate cortex, insulae, and thalamus.[61–63] One framework proposes medial (thalamus, anterior cingulate cortex, and prefrontal cortex) and lateral (primary and secondary somatosensory cortex) pain systems, and these have been investigated using functional imaging techniques.[64] Most functional imaging studies demonstrate activation in these structures with clinical or experimental pain, and recent reviews are available.[61,65] Recently, the amygdala,[61,66,67] basal ganglia,[61,68] and posterior parietal cortex[69] have also been implicated in central nervous system responses to pain.

It has been shown in migraine that the anterior cingulate cortex, frontal cortex, and visual and auditory association cortex are activated during acute attacks.[70] Similarly in cluster headache, cingulate cortex, insulae, prefrontal cortex, and basal ganglia are activated during pain.[59] The activation of these nonspecific areas during acute migraine and cluster headache is neither surprising nor unusual in pattern. How these areas relate to each other and the processing is unknown and will require challenging and technically difficult experiments to determine.

CENTRAL MODULATION OF TRIGEMINAL PAIN

A key observation, perhaps the crucial observation of functional imaging in migraine, has been that brain stem areas are active during pain and that after successful treatment this activation persists.[70] The activation corresponds with the brain region that Raskin et al.[71] initially reported and Veloso et al. confirmed,[72] to cause migraine-like headache in patients stimulated with electrodes implanted for pain control. Could these areas be pivotal in initiating or terminating the acute attack of migraine?

It has been shown in the experimental animal that stimulation of a discrete nucleus in the brain stem, nucleus locus coeruleus (the main central noradrenergic nucleus), reduces cerebral blood flow in a frequency-dependent manner[73] through an α_2-adrenoceptor–linked mechanism.[74] This reduction is maximal in the occipital cortex.[75] Although a 25% overall reduction in cerebral blood flow is seen, extracerebral vasodilatation occurs in parallel.[73] In addition, the main serotonin-containing nucleus in the brain stem, the midbrain dorsal raphe nucleus, can increase cerebral blood flow when activated.[9] We have recently seen that following stimulation of the SSS, Fos expression is increased in the ventrolateral periaqueductal grey matter (PAG) in the cat and monkey,[76] and we have also shown that stimulation of this region will inhibit SSS-evoked trigeminal neuronal activity in the cat.[77] The ventrolateral PAG would certainly have been included within the area of activation on the human neuroimaging studies outlined above, so its physiology and interactions with the trigeminovascular system are of particular interest. These aminergic brain stem neurons are an attractive site to host the basic defects in migraine and require detailed study and further human neuroimaging as we try to define the detail of the biology of migraine.

CONCLUSION

An understanding of the basic anatomy and physiology of the cranial circulation facilitates the assessment and management of patients with migraine. Physiologic processes clearly mature and change in childhood and adolescence, so it should not be a surprise that migraine evolves and changes, maturing to its adult form during adolescence. It seems likely that it is the brain control mechanisms that alter and mature, and perhaps this explains why the disease has the same flavor all through life but runs at different temperatures. It has become clear that migraine is not a vascular headache but that the trigeminovascular and parasympathetic innervation of the cranial circulation drives the vascular changes of migraine, which is in essence neurovascular in expression and a central nervous system disease process at its core. Migraine may be considered an episodic aminergic systems dysfunction with sensory-predominant consequences. Such a concept will drive new treatments, and an understanding of the basic anatomy and physiology of headache will aid clinical management at every level—from explaining the problem to the patient to initiating treatment.

REFERENCES

1. Lance JW, Goadsby PJ. Mechanism and Management of Headache. 6th ed. London: Butterworth-Heinemann, 1998.
2. Goadsby PJ. Bench to bedside: what have we learnt recently about headache? Curr Opin Neurol 1997;10:215–220.
3. Goadsby PJ, Silberstein SD. Headache. In: Asbury A, Marsden CD, eds. Blue Books in Practical Neurology: 17. New York: Butterworth-Heinemann, 1997.
4. McNaughton FL. The innervation of the intracranial blood vessels and the dural sinuses. In: Cobb S, Frantz AM, Penfield W, Riley HA, eds. The Circulation of the Brain and Spinal Cord. New York: Hafner Publishing, 1966, pp 178–200.
5. Arbab MA-R, Wiklund L, Svendgaard NA. Origin and distribution of cerebral vascular innervation from superior cervical, trigeminal and spinal ganglia investigated with retrograde and anterograde WGA-HRP tracing in the rat. Neuroscience 1986;19:695–708.
6. Uddman R, Edvinsson L, Ekman R, et al. Innervation of the feline cerebral vasculature by nerve fibers containing calcitonin gene-related peptide: trigeminal origin and co-existence with substance P. Neurosci Lett 1985;62:131–136.
7. Goadsby PJ, Edvinsson L, Ekman R. Release of vasoactive peptides in the extracerebral circulation of man and the cat during activation of the trigeminovascular system. Ann Neurol 1988;23:193–196.
8. Feindel W, Penfield W, McNaughton F. The tentorial nerves and localisation of intracranial pain in man. Neurology 1960;10:555–563.
9. Goadsby PJ, Zagami AS, Lambert GA. Neural processing of craniovascular pain: a synthesis of the central structures involved in migraine. Headache 1991;31:365–371.
10. Drummond PD, Lance JW. Extracranial vascular changes and the source of pain in migraine headache. Ann Neurol 1983;13:32–37.
11. Nichols FT, Mawad M, Mohr JP, et al. Focal headache during balloon inflation in the vertebral and basilar arteries. Headache 1993;33:87–89.
12. Nichols FT, Mawad M, Mohr JP, et al. Focal headache during balloon inflation in the internal carotid and middle cerebral arteries. Stroke 1990;21:555–559.

13. Martins IP, Baeta E, Paiva T, et al. Headaches during intracranial endovascular procedures: a possible model of vascular headache. Headache 1993;33: 227–233.

14. Moskowitz MA. Basic mechanisms in vascular headache. Neurol Clin 1990; 8:801–815.

15. Markowitz S, Saito K, Moskowitz MA. Neurogenically mediated leakage of plasma proteins occurs from blood vessels in dura mater but not brain. J Neurosci 1987;7:4129–4136.

16. Buzzi MG, Moskowitz MA. Evidence for 5-HT$_{1B/1D}$ receptors mediating the antimigraine effect of sumatriptan and dihydroergotamine. Cephalalgia 1991;11(4):165–168.

17. Buzzi MG, Sakas DE, Moskowitz MA. Indomethacin and acetylsalicylic acid block neurogenic plasma protein extravasation in rat dura mater. Eur J Pharmacol 1989;165:251–258.

18. Buzzi MG, Moskowitz MA. The antimigraine drug, sumatriptan (GR43175), selectively blocks neurogenic plasma extravasation from blood vessels in dura mater. Br J Pharmacol 1990;99:202–206.

19. Cutrer FM, Limmroth V, Waeber C, et al. New targets for antimigraine drug development. In: Goadsby PJ, Silberstein SD, eds. Headache. Philadelphia: Butterworth-Heinemann, 1997, pp 59–72.

20. Dimitriadou V, Buzzi MG, Moskowitz MA, Theoharides TC. Trigeminal sensory fiber stimulation induces morphological changes reflecting secretion in rat dura mater mast cells. Neuroscience 1991;44:97–112.

21. Dimitriadou V, Buzzi MG, Theoharides TC, Moskowitz MA. Ultrastructural evidence for neurogenically mediated changes in blood vessels of the rat dura mater and tongue following antidromic trigeminal stimulation. Neuroscience 1992;48:187–203.

22. Burstein R, Yamamura H, Malick A, Strassman AM. Chemical stimulation of the intracranial dura induces enhanced responses to facial stimulation in brain stem trigeminal neurons. J Neurophysiol 1998;79:964–982.

23. Strassman AM, Raymond SA, Burstein R. Sensitization of meningeal sensory neurons and the origin of headaches. Nature 1996;384:560–563.

24. May A, Shepheard S, Wessing A, et al. Retinal plasma extravasation can be evoked by trigeminal stimulation in rat but does not occur during migraine attacks. Brain 1998;121:1231–1237.

25. Diener HC. Substance-P antagonist RPR100893-201 is not effective in human migraine attacks. In: Olesen J, Tfelt-Hansen P, eds. Proceedings of the VIth International Headache Seminar. New York: Lippincott-Raven, 1996.

26. Goldstein DJ, Wang O, Saper JR, et al. Ineffectiveness of neurokinin-1 antagonist in acute migraine: a crossover study. Cephalalgia 1997;17:785–790.

27. Connor HE, Bertin L, Gillies S, et al. The GR205171 Clinical Study Group. Clinical evaluation of a novel, potent, CNS penetrating NK_1 receptor antagonist in the acute treatment of migraine. Cephalalgia 1998;18:392.

28. Norman B, Panebianco D, Block GA. A placebo-controlled, in-clinic study to explore the preliminary safety and efficacy of intravenous L-758,298 (a prodrug of the NK_1 receptor antagonist L-754,030) in the acute treatment of migraine. Cephalalgia 1998;18:407.

29. Roon K, Diener HC, Ellis P, et al. CP-122,288 blocks neurogenic inflammation, but is not effective in aborting migraine attacks: results of two controlled clinical studies. Cephalalgia 1997;17:245.

30. Earl NL, McDonald SA, Lowy MT, 4991W93 Investigator Group. Efficacy and tolerability of the neurogenic inflammation inhibitor, 4991W93, in the acute treatment of migraine. Cephalalgia 1999;19:357.

31. May A, Gijsman HJ, Wallnoefer A, et al. Endothelin antagonist bosentan blocks neurogenic inflammation, but is not effective in aborting migraine attacks. Pain 1996;67:375–378.

32. Data J, Britch K, Westergaard N, et al. A double-blind study of ganaxolone in the acute treatment of migraine headaches with or without an aura in premenopausal females. Headache 1998;38:380.

33. Goadsby PJ, Duckworth JW. Effect of stimulation of trigeminal ganglion on regional cerebral blood flow in cats. Am J Physiol 1987;253:R270–R274.

34. Goadsby PJ, Macdonald GJ. Extracranial vasodilation mediated by vasoactive intestinal polypeptide (VIP). Brain Res 1985;329:285–288.

35. Zagami AS, Goadsby PJ, Edvinsson L. Stimulation of the superior sagittal sinus in the cat causes release of vasoactive peptides. Neuropeptides 1990; 16:69–75.

36. Goadsby PJ, Edvinsson L, Ekman R. Vasoactive peptide release in the extracerebral circulation of humans during migraine headache. Ann Neurol 1990;28:183–187.

37. Gallai V, Sarchielli P, Floridi A, et al. Vasoactive peptides levels in the plasma of young migraine patients with and without aura assessed both interictally and ictally. Cephalalgia 1995;15:384–390.

38. Goadsby PJ, Edvinsson L. Human in vivo evidence for trigeminovascular activation in cluster headache. Brain 1994;117:427–434.

39. Fanciullacci M, Alessandri M, Figini M, et al. Increases in plasma calcitonin gene-related peptide from extracerebral circulation during nitroglycerin-induced cluster headache attack. Pain 1995;60:119–123.

40. Goadsby PJ, Edvinsson L. Neuropeptide changes in a case of chronic paroxysmal hemicrania—evidence for trigemino-parasympathetic activation. Cephalalgia 1996;16:448–450.

41. Knight YE, Edvinsson L, Goadsby PJ. Blockade of CGRP release after superior sagittal sinus stimulation in cat: a comparison of avitriptan and CP122,288. Neuropeptides 1999;33:41–46.

42. Knight YE, Connor HE, Edvinsson L, Goadsby PJ. Only 5HT$_{1B/1D}$ agonist doses of 4991W93 inhibit CGRP release in the cat. Cephalalgia 1999;19:401.

43. Nozaki K, Boccalini P, Moskowitz MA. Expression of c-fos-like immunoreactivity in brainstem after meningeal irritation by blood in the subarachnoid space. Neuroscience 1992;49:669–680.

44. Kaube H, Keay K, Hoskin KL, et al. Expression of c-Fos-like immunoreactivity in the caudal medulla and upper cervical spinal cord following stimulation of the superior sagittal sinus in the cat. Brain Res 1993;629:95–102.

45. Goadsby PJ, Hoskin KL. The distribution of trigeminovascular afferents in the nonhuman primate brain Macaca nemestrina: a c-fos immunocytochemical study. J Anat 1997;190:367–375.

46. Goadsby PJ, Zagami AS. Stimulation of the superior sagittal sinus increases metabolic activity and blood flow in certain regions of the brainstem and upper cervical spinal cord of the cat. Brain 1991;114:1001–1011.

47. Goadsby PJ, Hoskin KL, Knight YE. Stimulation of the greater occipital nerve increases metabolic activity in the trigeminal nucleus caudalis and cervical dorsal horn of the cat. Pain 1997;73:23–28.

48. Hoskin KL, Zagami A, Goadsby PJ. Stimulation of the middle meningeal artery leads to bilateral Fos expression in the trigeminocervical nucleus: a comparative study of monkey and cat. J Anat 1999;194:579–588.

49. Hoskin KL, Kaube H, Goadsby PJ. Central activation of the trigeminovascular pathway in the cat is inhibited by dihydroergotamine: a c-Fos and electrophysiology study. Brain 1996;119:249–256.

50. Kaube H, Hoskin KL, Goadsby PJ. Intravenous acetylsalicylic acid inhibits central trigeminal neurons in the dorsal horn of the upper cervical spinal cord in the cat. Headache 1993;33:541–550.

51. Kaube H, Hoskin KL, Goadsby PJ. Sumatriptan inhibits central trigeminal neurons only after blood-brain barrier disruption. Br J Pharmacol 1993;109:788–792.

52. Goadsby PJ, Hoskin KL. Differential effects of low dose CP122,288 and eletriptan on Fos expression due to stimulation of the superior sagittal sinus in the cat. Pain 1999;82:15–22.

53. Goadsby PJ, Knight YE. Naratriptan inhibits trigeminal neurons after intravenous administration through an action at the serotonin ($5HT_{1B/1D}$) receptors. Br J Pharmacol 1997;122:918–922.

54. Cumberbatch MJ, Hill RG, Hargreaves RJ. Differential effects of the $5HT_{1B/1D}$ receptor agonist naratriptan on trigeminal versus spinal nociceptive responses. Cephalalgia 1998;18:659–664.

55. Cumberbatch MJ, Hill RG, Hargreaves RJ. Rizatriptan has central antinociceptive effects against durally evoked responses. Eur J Pharmacol 1997;328:37–40.

56. Goadsby PJ, Hoskin KL. Inhibition of trigeminal neurons by intravenous administration of the serotonin (5HT)-1-D receptor agonist zolmitriptan (311C90): are brain stem sites a therapeutic target in migraine? Pain 1996; 67:355–359.

57. Zagami AS, Goadsby PJ. Stimulation of the superior sagittal sinus increases metabolic activity in cat thalamus. In: Rose FC, ed. New Advances in Headache Research: 2. London: Smith-Gordon and Co., 1991, pp 169–171.

58. Zagami AS, Lambert GA. Craniovascular application of capsaicin activates nociceptive thalamic neurons in the cat. Neurosci Lett 1991;121:187–190.

59. May A, Bahra A, Buchel C, et al. Hypothalamic activation in cluster headache attacks. Lancet 1998;351:275–278.

60. May A, Bahra A, Buchel C, et al. Functional magnetic resonance imaging in spontaneous attacks of SUNCT: short-lasting neuralgiform headache with conjunctival injection and tearing. Ann Neurol 1999;46:791–793.

61. Derbyshire SWG, Jones AKP, Gyulai F, et al. Pain processing during three levels of noxious stimulation produces differential patterns of central activity. Pain 1997;73:431–445.

62. Jones AK, Brown WD, Friston KJ, et al. Cortical and subcortical localization of response to pain in man using positron emission tomography. Proc R Soc Lond Biol Sci 1991;244:39–44.

63. Melzack R, Casey KL. Sensory, motivational and central control determinants of pain. In: Kenshalo DR, ed. The Skin Senses. Springfield Il: CC Thomas, 1968, pp 423–439.

64. Jones AK, Qi LY, Fujirawa T, et al. In vivo distribution of opioid receptors in man in relation to the cortical projections of the medial and lateral pain systems measured with positron emission tomography. Neurosci Lett 1991;126:25–28.

65. Chen AC. Human brain measures of clinical pain: a review. II. Tomographic imaging. Pain 1993;54:133–144.

66. Bernard JF, Huang GF, Besson JM. Nucleus centralis of the amygdala and the globus pallidus ventralis: electrophysiological evidence for an involvement in pain processes. J Neurophysiol 1992;68:551–569.

67. Hsieh JC, Stahle-Backdahl M, Hagermark O, et al. Traumatic nociceptive pain activates the hypothalamus and the periacqueductal gray: a positron emission tomography study. Pain 1996;64:303–314.

68. Chudler EH, Dong WK. The role of the basal ganglia in nociception and pain. Pain 1995;60:33–38.

69. Dong WK, Hayashi T, Roberts VJ, et al. Behavioral outcome of posterior parietal cortex injury in the monkey. Pain 1996;64:579–587.

70. Weiller C, May A, Limmroth V, et al. Brain stem activation in spontaneous human migraine attacks. Nat Med 1995;1:658–660.

71. Raskin NH, Hosobuchi Y, Lamb S. Headache may arise from perturbation of brain. Headache 1987;27:416–420.

72. Veloso F, Kumar K, Toth C. Headache secondary to deep brain implantation. Headache 1998;38:507–515.

73. Goadsby PJ, Lambert GA, Lance JW. Differential effects on the internal and external carotid circulation of the monkey evoked by locus coeruleus stimulation. Brain Res 1982;249:247–254.

74. Goadsby PJ, Lambert GA, Lance JW. The mechanism of cerebrovascular vasoconstriction in response to locus coeruleus stimulation. Brain Res 1985;326:213–217.

75. Goadsby PJ, Duckworth JW. Low frequency stimulation of the locus coeruleus reduces regional cerebral blood flow in the spinalized cat. Brain Res 1989;476:71–77.

76. Hoskin KL, Bulmer DCE, Jonkman A, Goadsby PJ. The role of the periaqueductal gray (PAG) in the pathogenesis of migraine. Cephalalgia 1999;19:314.

77. Knight YE, Goadsby PJ. Brainstem stimulation inhibits trigeminal neurons in the cat. Cephalalgia 1999;19:315.

Chapter 5

MIGRAINE, MIGRAINE VARIANTS, AND OTHER PRIMARY HEADACHE SYNDROMES

Donald W. Lewis and Paul Winner

Children with headache are brought to medical attention by their parents primarily for reassurance that the headaches are not a sign of a brain tumor or serious illness. A thorough history, physical examination, and when appropriate, diagnostic testing will enable the practitioner to distinguish primary headaches from those of a secondary etiology. The less common primary headache syndromes, as well as secondary headache disorders, can provoke considerable anxiety in the patients and their parents.

The evaluation of the child, especially under the age of 10 years, requires creative techniques as well as input from the parents in order to obtain a complete history. It is important to determine whether there is more than one type of headache experienced by the child. The number of days missed from school can help determine the frequency, severity, and disability of the headaches.

MIGRAINE

Migraine, an episodic sick headache, is characterized by recurrent episodes of throbbing head pain of variable intensity, duration, and frequency with associated nausea and vomiting, as well as photophobia and/or phonophobia. The attacks are separated by pain-free intervals. The International Headache Society (IHS) provides explicit criteria for the diagnosis of migraine (Table 5–1).[1] However, the IHS criteria do not characterize headaches in children separately and lack sensitivity in this population.[2–4]

Valquist was one of the first to propose the definition of migraine as paroxysmal headache separated by pain-free intervals and accompanied by at least two of the following four features: visual aura, nausea, unilateral pain, and family history of migraine.[5,6] Bille reinforced the intermittent nature of the headache but required three of the same four accompanying features.[7] In 1976, Prensky redefined migraine as paroxysmal headache, expanding the associated symptoms to three of six including aura, abdominal pain, unilateral location, throbbing quality, relief with sleep, and family history of migraine.[8,9]

Many authors have challenged these established criteria. Millichap found the throbbing quality an unreliable feature.[10] Gladstein and others have questioned the unilateral location as being uncommon in childhood migraine wherein a bifrontal or retro-orbital localization is more frequently reported.[2,4,11] Seshia et al. examined the applicability of IHS criteria to childhood migraine and found three factors that limit its usefulness[4]: inability of the child or guardian to provide adequate description of the headache,[5] inability to meet the criterion for minimum duration (2 hours),[12] and low incidence of associated features (location, quality of pain, aggravation by exercise).[4]

Table 5–1   IHS Classification

Pediatric Migraine Without Aura	Pediatric Migraine With Aura*
Diagnostic Criteria	Diagnostic Criteria
A. At least five attacks fulfilling B–D	A. At least two attacks fulfilling B
B. Headache attack lasting 2–48 hours	B. At least three of the following: 1. One or more fully reversible aura symptoms indicating focal cortical and/or brain stem dysfunction
C. Headache has at least two of the following: 1. Unilateral location 2. Pulsating quality	2. At least one aura developing gradually over more than 4 minutes or two or more symptoms occurring in succession
3. Moderate to severe intensity 4. Aggravation by routine physical activity	3. No auras lasting more than 60 minutes 4. Headache follows less than 60 minutes
D. During headache, at least one of the following: 1. Nausea and/or vomiting 2. Photophobia or phonophobia	

*Idiopathic recurring disorder; headache usually lasts 2 to 48 hours in patients less than 15 years of age.
Adapted from: Classification and diagnostic criteria for headache disorders, cranial neuralgia and facial pain. Headache Classification Committee of the International Headache Society. Cephalalgia 1988;8(Suppl 7):1–96.

A revised classification of symptoms based on the IHS criteria (Table 5–2) is currently being tested.[13] Both the IHS and the new revised IHS-R (HIS-R) criteria require multiple headache attacks. The first migraine attack cannot always be differentiated from symptomatic headache due to, for example, infection, concussion, or neoplasm. In children, especially younger children, the duration of headache may be as little as 1 hour. Migraine headaches are often bilateral (bifrontal or bitemporal) particularly in the younger child.[4,13–15] Headaches occurring in the occipital area are more unusual and may have an organic cause. Careful questioning of the parents and a little persistence is crucial in finding out what the child does and how the child's routine is altered during headaches. For example, will the child watch television during headaches? Does the headache interfere with the child's social activities and academic performance?

The associated symptoms of migraine are an integral part of the disorder and are essential to diagnosis. They include photophobia, phonophobia, nausea, and vomiting. Nausea occurs in most migrainous patients, whether child or adult. Vomiting occurs in both, but in children it may occur earlier in the headache episode. Adults often experience some pho-

Table 5–2   Proposed Revised IHS Classification

Pediatric Migraine Without Aura	Pediatric Migraine With Aura*
Diagnostic Criteria	*Diagnostic Criteria*
A. At least five attacks fulfilling B–D	A. At least two attacks fulfilling B
B. Headache attack lasting 1–48 hours	B. At least three of the following: 1. One or more fully reversible aura symptoms indicating focal cortical and/or brain stem dysfunction
C. Headache has at least two of the following: 1. Bilateral location (frontal/temporal) or unilateral location 2. Pulsating quality 3. Moderate to severe intensity 4. Aggravation by routine physical activity	2. At least one aura developing gradually over more than 4 minutes or two or more symptoms occurring in succession 3. No auras lasting more than 60 minutes 4. Headache follows less than 60 minutes
D. During headache, at least one of the following: 1. Nausea and/or vomiting 2. Photophobia and/or phonophobia	

*Idiopathic recurring disorder; headache usually lasts 1 to 48 hours.
Adapted from: Winner P, Martinez W, Mate L, Bello L. Classification of pediatric migraine: proposed revisions of the IHS criteria. Headache 1995;35:407–410.

tophobia and phonophobia, whereas children are more likely to experience one of these symptoms.[14]

Migraine without Aura (Common Migraine)

Migraine without aura is the most frequent form, estimated to account for 60 to 85% of all migraine. A recent meta-analysis of adolescents who meet IHS criteria for migraine (n = 1,932) reported 67% with migraine without aura and an additional 19% noting both migraine with and without aura.[16]

Parents will often recognize early prodromal features: mood changes (euphoria to depression), irritability, lethargy, yawning, food cravings, or increased thirst. Perhaps the most frequent heralding feature is a change in behavior or withdrawal from activity.

The older, more verbally sophisticated children will report periodic headaches localized to the frontal or temporal regions, occasionally unilaterally, and describe a pounding, pulsing, throbbing quality to the pain. In a recent adolescent demographic analysis, 58% reported unilateral pain, and 88% recorded that the pain was aggravated by activity.[16] Photophobia and/or phonophobia are common (80% recorded in this same study) and often prompt the child to seek a quiet, dark place to rest or even to sleep, as sleep often produces significant relief. The characteristic features are shown in Table 5–3.

Migraine headache typically last hours to days (1 to 48 hours), but it does not generally occur more frequently than six to eight times per month. More than 8 to 10 events per month must warrant consideration of alternative diagnoses such as organic causes or chronic daily headache syndromes.[17,18] Migraine in adolescents is more commonly reported on Mondays (20%), followed by Tuesdays (16%), and Wednesdays (16%).[16]

Nausea, vomiting, and abdominal pain may be intense and are often the most disabling features. For example, a student with headache may be able to stay in the classroom, but the onset of nausea or vomiting will require the student to visit the school nurse. Nausea was reported in 60% of adolescents, whereas vomiting was recorded in only 5% of the migraines.[16]

The time of day when the headache occurs tends to shift through childhood. Younger children will complain in the afternoon, after school.

Table 5–3   Migraine: Associated Symptoms

Prodromal (hours or days in advance)	Autonomic symptoms
Mood changes	Nausea, vomiting, anorexia
Irritability	Periumbilical abdominal pain
Euphoria	Diarrhea
Increased thirst	Pallor
Increase urination	Phonophobia/photophobia
Fluid retention	Desire to sleep
Food cravings (high carbohydrate food)	Cool extremities
Yawning, sighing	Periorbital discoloration
The headache	"Goose flesh"
Gradual onset	Increased or decreased blood pressure
Escalates over minutes to hours	Syncope
Lasts 2–72 hours	Miscellaneous
Frontal, bitemporal, retro-orbital, unilateral	Motion sickness
Pounding, pulsing, throbbing	Sleep walking
Intensity increased by activity	Recurrent abdominal pain

The younger teenagers will frequently begin to report their headaches about lunchtime, maybe precipitated by the chaos of the school cafeteria with its combination of bright lights, loud noise, and peer pressures. Older teens will acquire the more adult patterns of morning headache. The morning occurrence frequently raises suspicion of space-occupying lesions. In adolescents, 6 am to 6 pm accounts for 73% of reported migraines.[16]

Although these symptoms can be clearly related by more mature children, the younger or developmentally challenged patients may be unable to verbalize these complains. Parents will report repeated cyclic events of quiet, withdrawn behavior, pallor, regurgitation, vomiting, and desire to rest. These features are particularly noticeable in the active toddler who will halt play, withdraw to a quiet spot, and vomit or sleep. These episodes may prompt investigation for epilepsy, gastroesophageal reflux, or hydrocephalus, when, in fact, they may represent migraine. The common thread between these events in the very young child and the non-communicative child is the stereotypic, cyclic pattern of pallor, vomiting, and withdrawn behavior. These stereotypic episodes should prompt consideration of migraine in the pre- or early verbal child.[19]

Migraine with Aura (Classic Migraine)

Approximately 14 to 30% of children and adolescents will report visual disturbances, distortions, or obscuration before or as the headache begins. The aura is an inconsistent feature in childhood and a less reliable heralding phenomenon than in adult migraineurs. Some children will present with a complaint of seeing spots, balloons, colors, or rainbows, but usually the symptom must be elicited by asking very pointed questions, for example "Do you have spots, colors, lights, or dots in your eyes as you get a headache?" Hachinski et al.'s classic report of children's visual symptomatology found three dominant visual phenomena: binocular visual impairment with scotoma (77%), distortion or hallucinations (16%), and monocular visual impairment or scotoma (7%).[20]

The diagnosis of migraine with aura requires the patient to present with one or more fully reversible neurologic symptoms including visual, motor, or sensory symptoms. The symptoms help to distinguish migraine from a progressive, organic disorder that requires further diagnostic assessment. The aura should develop gradually over at least 4 minutes. It usually lasts 20 to 30 minutes but may last as long as 60 minutes.[1] If the aura is short in duration or rapid in onset, an alternate paroxysmal event may be the cause.

The onset of the visual aura, characterized by sudden images and complicated visual perceptions, should prompt consideration of benign occipital epilepsy, even if followed by headache. Bizarre visual phenomena may be seen in the "Alice in Wonderland" syndrome. Transient visual obscuration, to the point of complete blindness, is also a variable feature of pseudotumor cerebri.

Migrainous patients have been reported to have nonspecific electroencephalographic abnormalities. Some of the abnormalities are now believed to be normal variants such as 14 and 6 phantom spike; others are felt to be a benign rolandic pattern, which often does not require treatment.[21,22]

MIGRAINE VARIANTS

On occasion, clinical forms of migraine present with dramatic neurologic signs, such as hemiparesis, ataxia, acute confusional states, ophthalmoparesis, or vertigo. These clinical entities are termed "migraine variants."

The abrupt appearance of such focal and ominous neurologic signs accompanying an excruciating headache with vomiting must, however, initially raise concerns toward life-threatening neurologic emergencies, such as intracranial hemorrhage, brain tumor, hydrocephalus, central nervous system (CNS) infection, or intoxication. Only after a careful history, physical and neurologic examination, and appropriate neurodiagnostic studies can the diagnosis of migraine variant be comfortably entertained. All represent diagnoses of exclusion.

Traditionally, the migraine variants have been thought to occur as a result of vasoconstriction with resultant focal hypoperfusion and transient deficits due to ischemia within a specific cerebral arterial distribution. In theory then, oligemia within the vertebrobasilar artery territory would cause the variety of symptoms associated with basilar migraine (i.e., ataxia, vertigo, diplopia) or middle cerebral artery oligemia, producing contralateral hemiparesis with language disorders in hemiplegic migraine.

The pathogenesis of the migraine variants is clearly not that simple. As understanding of migraine evolves, we must re-examine the mechanisms responsible for the migraine variants. Current evidence suggests a primary neuronal initiation to the cascade of events leading to migraine attacks, as discussed in Chapter 4, "Migraine Pathophysiology." In migraine with aura, transient focal deficits, usually visual symptoms, are the result of a wave of depolarization migrating across the visual cortex and/or regional oligemia caused by a neuropeptide-mediated, sterile, neurogenic inflammation.

The transient deficits of the migraine variants are now thought to result from the same process, as evidenced by inclusion of the variants within the spectrum of migraine with aura. From the clinical perspective, there are frequently shared or overlapping clinical features with many of the variants, and this observation also supports the concept of a common pathophysiology. Still incompletely explained under this postulate, however, are the cranial nerve signs associated with ophthalmoplegic and basilar migraine.

The classification system for migraine has evolved from the traditional grouping (Table 5–4) to that currently accepted by the IHS

Table 5–4　Migraine Classification: Traditional

Common migraine

Classic migraine

Complicated migraine
  Basilar artery migraine
  Ophthalmoplegic migraine
  Confusional migraine
  "Alice in Wonderland" syndrome
  Hemiplegic migraine

Migraine variants
  Benign paroxysmal vertigo
  Cyclic vomiting
  ?Paroxysmal torticollis

?Abdominal migraine

(Table 5–5).[1] As mentioned, inclusion of hemiplegic and basilar migraine variants within the spectrum of migraine with aura reflects the contemporary view of their pathogenesis. The IHS system fails to include the clinical entities of confusional migraine and cyclic vomiting, but both will be addressed in this chapter. Also omitted by the IHS classification is the

Table 5–5　IHS Migraine Classification

1.1 Migraine without aura (common migraine)

1.2 Migraine with aura (classic migraine)
  1.2.1 Migraine with typical aura
  1.2.2 Migraine with prolonged aura
  1.2.3 Familial hemiplegic migraine
  1.2.4 Basilar migraine
  1.2.5 Migraine aura without headache
  1.2.6 Migraine with acute onset aura

1.3 Ophthalmoplegic migraine

1.4 Retinal migraine

1.5 Childhood periodic syndromes that may be precursors to or associated with migraine
  1.5.1 Benign paroxysmal vertigo
  1.5.2 Alternating hemiplegia of childhood

Adapted from: Classification and diagnostic criteria for headache disorders, cranial neuralgia and facial pain. Headache Classification Committee of the International Headache Society. Cephalalgia 1988;8(Suppl 7):1–96.

"Alice in Wonderland" syndrome, which most likely represents an unusual form of visual aura with distortions, illusions, micropsia, and macropsia.

Familial Hemiplegic Migraine

Familial hemiplegic migraine (FHM) (IHS classification 1.2.3) is an uncommon autosomal dominant form of migraine headache in which the aura has a "stroke-like" quality producing some degree of hemiparesis. The nosology is somewhat misleading since there is actually a wide diversity of symptoms and signs that can accompany this migraine variant beyond motor deficits (Table 5–6). Barlow proposed the more appropriate term "hemisyndrome migraine" to emphasize the diversity of associated symptoms, but this has not received broad acceptance.[23] The IHS criteria clearly requires that "some degree of hemiparesis" must be present, so the term will likely persist.[1]

A series of recent exciting discoveries into the molecular genetics of FHM have broadened our understanding of the fundamental mechanisms of migraine and demonstrated the overlap with other paroxysmal disorders such as acetazolamide-responsive episodic ataxia.[24] Genetic linkage to chromosome 19p13 has been identified in half of the known FHM pedigrees, and more recently, a separate pedigree with linkage to chromosome 1q31 has been reported.[25,26] The chromosomal 19 defect produces a missense mutation in a neuronal calcium channel gene providing compelling evidence that FHM represents a channelopathy.[25] These discoveries have

Table 5–6   Hemiplegic or Hemisyndrome Migraine Signs and Symptoms

Motor
  Hemiplegia, hemiparesis, monoplegia, monoparesis
Sensory
  Hemidysesthesia, hemihypesthesia, hemianesthesia, cheiro-oral or digitolingual dysesthesias
Confusion
Dysphasia, aphasia, dysarthria
Visual
  Hemianopia, quadrantanopia

Adapted from: Lewis DW. Migraine and migraine variant in childhood and adolescence. Semin Pediatr Neurol 1995;2:127–143.

revolutionized our understanding of migraine and may open new territory for pharmacologic interventions.

From the clinical perspective, hemiplegic migraine is characterized by transient (hours to days) episodes of focal neurologic deficits that precede the headache phase by 30 to 60 minutes but, occasionally, extend well beyond the headache itself. The headache is often, but not invariably, contralateral to the focal deficit.

The appearance of acute focal neurologic deficits in the setting of headache in a child necessitates vigorous investigation for disorders such as those listed in Table 5–7. Neuroimaging, such as magnetic resonance imaging (MRI) and magnetic resonance angiography (MRA) and electroencephalography (EEG) may be indicated. Investigations for embolic sources or hypercoagulable states are likewise appropriate.

*M*itochondrial *e*ncephalomyopathy, *l*actic *a*cidosis, and *s*troke-like attack (MELAS) warrants particular attention in the differential diagnosis of hemiplegic migraine because of the high frequency of migraine-like headache in MELAS patients. MELAS is caused by a point mutation in the mitochondrial DNA (mtDNA) (A→G @ 3243mtDNA) and clinically characterized by episodes of focal neurologic deficits with variable MRI changes that do not, generally, respect vascular territories. Although there is some overlap of symptoms with hemiplegic migraine, children with MELAS also have muscle weakness and atrophy, dementia, and epilepsy. Serum lactic acid levels are usually quite elevated and the diagnosis is confirmed by specific mtDNA testing.

Alternating Hemiplegia of Childhood

Alternating hemiplegia of childhood (AHC) (IHS classification 1.5.2) is a rare and fascinating syndrome that has traditionally been considered a variant of hemiplegic migraine.

Initial symptoms begin before 18 months of life. Affected children have attacks of paralysis: hemiparesis, monoparesis, diparesis, ophthalmoparesis, and bulbar paralysis, which may be accompanied by variable tone changes (e.g., flaccid, spastic, rigid). A variety of paroxysmal involuntary movements, including chorea, athetosis, dystonia, nystagmus, and respiratory irregularities (hyperpnea), can be seen. The attacks of paralysis can be brief (minutes) or prolonged (days) and potentially life threatening during periods of bulbar paralysis. Curiously, the attacks generally subside following sleep. Affected children are frequently developmentally challenged.[27,28]

The link to migraine is based on the presence of a high incidence of migraine in the families of affected children and on cerebral blood flow data, which suggest a migrainous mechanism.

Table 5–7   Acute Focal Deficits in Childhood

Hemiplegic migraine

Cerebral infarction

    Embolic infarction: cardiac, arterial dissection

    Thrombotic infarction

Hypercoagulable states—protein S or C deficiency

    Hemoglobinopathy, sickle cell anemia

    Hyperviscous states, leukemia

    Thrombocytosis, dehydration

Vasculitis, systemic lupus erythematosus

Cerebral hemorrhage

    Vascular malformation, cavernous angioma, aneurysm, post-traumatic hemorrhage

    Hypertensive hemorrhage (renal disease, substance abuse—cocaine)

Metabolic deficit

Homocystinuria

    MELAS

Infection

    Brain abscess, epidural empyema

    Encephalitis, meningitis

    Septic thrombosis (cavernous sinus, sagittal sinus, cortical veins)

Neoplastic deficit

    Tumor (astrocytoma, ganglioglioma, meningioma, ependymoma)

    Metastasis (sarcoma, lymphoma)

Post-ictal deficit (Todd's paralysis)

Demyelinative disorder

    Multiple sclerosis

    Acute disseminated encephalomyelitis

MELAS = mitochondrial encephalomyopathy, lactic acidosis, and stroke-like attacks.
Adapted from: Lewis DW. Migraine and migraine variant in childhood and adolescence. Semin Pediatr Neurol 1995;2:127–143.

In 1997, an international workshop was conducted to address the various hypotheses surrounding AHC, and the proceedings have been reviewed by Rho and Chugani.[29] Proposed mechanisms include channelopathy, mitochondrial cytopathy, and cerebrovascular dysfunction, although channelopathy seems to be the most likely hypothesis. The calcium channel blocker flunarizine can be remarkably effective in reducing attack frequency and severity.

This somewhat bizarre entity warrants aggressive evaluation for vascular disorders, inborn errors of metabolism, mitochondrial encephalomyopathies, or epileptic variants.

Basilar Migraine

Also known as "basilar artery," "vertebrobasilar," or "Bickerstaff migraine," basilar migraine (BM) (IHM classification 1.2.4) is the most frequent of the complicated migraine variants and is estimated to represent 3 to 19% of all migraine.[30–33] This wide range of frequency relates to the rigorousness of the definition. Some authors include any headache with dizziness to be within the spectrum of BM, whereas others require the presence of clear signs and symptoms of posterior fossa involvement before establishing this diagnosis. The IHS criteria require two or more symptoms (Table 5–8) and emphasize bulbar and bilateral sensorimotor features.[1]

The mean age of onset of BM tends to be 7 years, although the clinical entity probably appears as early as 12 to 18 months as episodic pallor, clumsiness, and vomiting (see the section in this chapter on benign paroxysmal vertigo).

Affected children will have attacks of intense dizziness, vertigo, visual disturbances, ataxia, and diplopia. These early transient features last minutes to an hour and are then followed by the headache phase. But unlike headaches with the more typical frontal or temporal location, this headache may be occipital in location. The quality of the pain may be difficult for the child to describe, and terms such as "pulsing" or "throbbing" may not be used. A small subset of children with BM will have their posterior fossa symptoms after the headache phase is well established.

The pathogenesis of BM is not well understood. Although focal cortical processes, oligemia, or depolarization can explain the deficits in hemi-

Table 5–8   Basilar Migraine: Signs and Symptoms

Sign/Symptom	Percentage
Vertigo	73
Nausea or vomiting	30–50
Ataxia	43–50
Visual field deficits	43
Diplopia	30
Tinnitus	13
Hearing loss*	—
Confusion	20
Dysarthria*	—
Weakness (hemiplegia, quadriplegia, diplegia)	20
Syncope*	—

*No incidence figures available.
Adapted from: Bickerstaff ER. Basilar artery migraine. Lancet 1961;1:15–17; Lapkin ML, Golden GS. Basilar artery migraine. A review of 30 cases. Am J Dis Child 1978;132:278–281; Barlow CF. Headaches and migraine in childhood. Clin Dev Med 1984;91:103–109; Golden GS, French JH. Basilar artery migraine in young children. Pediatrics 1975;56:722–726; Lewis DW. Migraine and migraine variant in childhood and adolescence. Semin Pediatr Neurol 1995;2:127–143.

plegic migraine, the posterior fossa signs of BM are more problematic. A single case report of a 25-year-old woman with BM exists wherein transcranial Doppler and single photon emission computed tomography (SPECT) were performed through the course of a BM attack. These data suggest decreased posterior cerebral artery perfusion through the aura phase at a time when the patient was experiencing transient bilateral blindness and ataxia.[34]

The sudden appearance of diplopia, vertigo, and vomiting must prompt consideration of disorders within the posterior fossa such as arteriovenous malformations, cavernous angiomas, tumors (i.e., medulloblastoma, ependymoma, brain stem glioma), congenital malformations (i.e., Chiari, Dandy-Walker), or vertebrobasilar insufficiency (i.e., vertebral dissection or thrombosis). Acute labyrinthitis or positional vertigo can mimic BM. Platybasia or basilar impression can infrequently present with unusual headache symptomatology. Complex partial seizures and drug ingestions must be considered at any age. Rarely, metabolic diseases, such as Hartnup disease, hyperammonemias (i.e., urea cycle or organic acidemias), or disorders of pyruvate/lactate metabolism may present with episodic vertigo, but these inborn errors of metabolism usually have some degree of altered consciousness, even coma.

Ophthalmoplegic Migraine

Ophthalmoplegic migraine (OM) (IHS classification 1.3) is one of the most dramatic and clinically challenging migraine variants and, fortunately, one of the least common. Available epidemiologic data suggest an annual incidence of 0.7 per million.[35] The two key features are ophthalmoparesis and headache, although the headache may be mild or a nondescript retro-orbital discomfort. Whereas verbally sophisticated school-aged children may describe blurred vision or diplopia, young children may simply rub their eyes. Attacks of OM have been reported during infancy, as early as 5 to 7 months of age.[36]

Ptosis, adduction defects, and skew deviations are the common objective findings.

The time course of OM is quite different from that of the more commonly encountered migraine variants. Symptoms and signs of oculomotor dysfunction may appear well into the headache phase, rather than herald the headache. The signs may persist for days or even weeks after the headache has resolved.

The oculomotor nerve, or its divisions, are the most frequently involved, but pupillary involvement is inconsistent and controversial. In our experience of three cases, all had pupillary involvement. Some authors report pupillary involvement in only one-third of patients.[37] The third nerve involvement may be incomplete, with partial deficits in both the inferior and superior division of the third nerve. Abduction defects, due to abducens involvement, are the second most frequent reported variant of OM, and trochlear nerve is the least common.

The mechanism of OM is openly debated. The primary theories suggest ischemic, compressive, or inflammatory processes.[16] Lack of pupillary involvement argues for an ischemic mechanism, whereas a higher incidence of pupillary involvement weighs toward a compressive mechanism. Alternatively, recent reports have questioned whether OM may be an inflammatory process within the spectrum of Tolosa-Hunt syndrome, particularly given the steroid responsiveness of many patients.[38] Furthermore, high resolution neuroimaging has shown a reversible enhancement and even thickening of the oculomotor nerve during attacks, which lends further credence to an inflammatory mechanism.[39]

The differential diagnosis for OM is shown in Table 5–9. Aneurysm or mass lesion in or around the orbital apex and parasellar region must be aggressively sought. Imaging with MRI or MRA is usually indicated. The performance of angiography is recommended by some authors and cautioned against by others because of the theoretic risk of vasospasm with contrast agents in migraine patients.

In those children with external ophthalmoparesis, test doses of edrophonium are indicated to exclude ocular myasthenia.

Repeated attacks of OM can lead to permanent deficits; therefore acute treatment with steroids and prophylactic treatment must be considered.

Retinal Migraine

Also referred to as "ocular," "ophthalmic," or "anterior visual pathway migraine," retinal migraine (IHS classification 1.4) is extremely uncom-

Table 5–9   Ophthalmoparesis in Childhood

Ophthalmoplegic migraine
Head trauma
Thyroid disease (Graves' disease)
Myasthenia gravis, ocular myasthenia
Chronic progressive external ophthalmoplegia (Kearns-Sayre syndrome)
Miller Fisher syndrome variant of Guillain-Barré syndrome
Orbital pseudotumor
Tolosa-Hunt syndrome
Sarcoidosis
Cerebral aneurysms (intracavernous carotid artery, posterior communicating)
Cavernous sinus thrombosis
Orbital tumors (lymphoma, sarcoma)
Orbital abscess
Postinfections
Metabolic—diabetic, branched-chain aminoacidopathy, nonketotic hyperglycinemia
Idiopathic opthalmoparesis

Lewis DW. Migraine and migraine variant in childhood and adolescence. Semin Pediatr Neurol 1995;2:127–143.

mon in children and usually seen in young adults. Unlike the descending curtain-like onset of amaurosis fugax, retinal migraine causes patients to experience brief (seconds to < 60 minutes), sudden, monocular blackouts or "grayouts" or bright, blinding episodes (photopsia) of visual disturbance before, after, or during the headache. A 60-minute interval between visual symptom and headache may occur. As with ophthalmoplegic migraine, the pain is often described as retro-orbital and ipsilateral to the visual disturbance.

Examination of the fundus during an attack may disclose constriction of the retinal veins and arteries with retinal pallor. An occasional patient may suffer a significant visual sequela (e.g., scotoma, altitudinal defects, monocular blindness) presumably due to vasoconstriction with retinal infarction. Using a rat model, May et al., demonstrated the evolution of a sterile neurogenic inflammation in both the retina and dura following stimulation of the trigeminal ganglion but were unable to view the same phenomena in human retina in acute migraine.[40]

Although the patient population with retinal migraine is generally much younger than those who experience amaurosis fugax from atheromatous carotid disease, evaluation for hypercoagualable states, embolic sources, and vascular disruption (carotid dissection) must be considered.

"Alice in Wonderland" Syndrome

Bizarre visual illusions and spatial distortions occasionally precede headaches. Similar to Alice's visual distortions following the eating of a mushroom in the classic book *Through the Looking Glass*, affected children will describe visual distortions before or as the headache is beginning. The children may describe bizarre or vivid visual illusions such as micropsia, where objects appear smaller; macropsia, where objects appear larger; metamorphopsia, where objects (such as faces) appear distorted; and teleopsia, where objects appear far away.

Anecdotally, the children are not confused or frightened by these illusions and are able to relate the experience with detail. This unusual visual symptomatology is best considered as migraine with aura, although historically, "Alice in Wonderland" syndrome is included as a distinct variant. This type of visual-perceptual abnormality has been reported with infectious mononucleosis, complex partial seizures (particularly benign occipital epilepsy), and drug ingestions.

Confusional Migraine

In 1970, Gascon and Barlow reported a series of children, ages 8 to 16 years, with acute confusional states, lasting 4 to 24 hours, associated with agitation and aphasia as a presenting feature of juvenile migraine.[41] Ehyai and Fenichel later introduced the term "acute confusional migraine."[42] Subsequent reports have broadened the clinical phenomenology to include blindness, paresthesias, hemiparesis, and amnesia. Amnesia can be such a prominent feature that Jensen proposed the term "transient global amnesia of childhood," but amnesia is just part of the spectrum.[43]

Affected patients, usually boys, become agitated, restless, disoriented, and occasionally, combative for minutes to hours. Once consciousness has returned to baseline, the patients will describe an inability to communicate, frustration, confusion, loss of orientation to time, and they may not recall a headache phase at all. A strong family history of migraine is elicited in 75% of patients.

There is a clear link to head trauma in many cases.[44] The term "footballer's migraine" is applied in Europe when a soccer player, after heading the ball, develops an acute confusional state with headache. Similar phenomena may follow other causes of minor head injury. This should be viewed within the spectrum of trauma-triggered migraine.

As mentioned in the introduction to this chapter, there is a great deal of overlap between the various migraine variants, none more so than confusional migraine in which features of hemiplegic and basilar migraine may coexist. Perhaps this entity of confusional migraine is, in fact, a hybrid and should best be included within the spectrum of either basilar of hemiplegic migraine, depending on which symptoms predominate in individual patients. Those with aphasia, hemiparesis, and confusion are likely hemiplegic, and those with bilateral blindness, vertigo, and confusion are classified as basilar migraine.

Acute confusional states in children and adolescents warrant aggressive investigation for encephalitis, brain abscess, drug intoxication, cerebrovascular disease, vasculitis, or metabolic encephalopathies.[45] Particular attention must be focused on the possibility of complex partial seizures or post-ictal states.

Childhood Periodic Syndromes

Two clinical entities, formerly known as "migraine equivalents," are included by the IHS in childhood periodic syndromes: benign paroxysmal vertigo (BPV) and alternating hemiplegia of childhood (discussed earlier in this chapter). Benign paroxysmal torticollis (BPT), cyclic vomiting syndrome (CVS), and abdominal migraine are best discussed in this category also.

Benign Paroxysmal Vertigo

Benign paroxysmal vertigo is quite common, although incidence figures are lacking. Typically, affected young children (median 18 months) will be struck by a sudden unsteadiness on their feet. They will anxiously grab onto a nearby table, chair, or adult for stability or fall to the ground. Consciousness will not be lost but astute observers may notice nystagmus. Vomiting may be vigorous. The spells usually last minutes, and afterward the children will sleep. On awakening, they return to their normal baseline. The spells will occur in clusters over several days, then subside for weeks or months.[46,47]

These spells probably represent the early evolution of basilar migraine and the differential diagnosis would be similar. During a long-term follow-up of seven cases, Lanzi et al. reported five of seven BPV cases spontaneously resolved and six of seven patients later developed migraine and other migraine-related symptoms. The authors suggest that BPV can be interpreted as a migraine precursor.[48]

Benign Paroxysmal Torticollis

Benign paroxysmal torticollis is a rare paroxysmal dyskinesia characterized by attacks of head tilt alone or accompanied by vomiting and ataxia which may last hours to days.[49] Other torsional or dystonic features, including truncal or pelvic posturing, were described by Chutorian.[50] Attacks first manifest during infancy between 2 and 8 months of age.

The original descriptions of BPT by Snyder suggested a form of labyrinthitis and demonstrated abnormal vestibular reflexes.[51]

The link to migraine is twofold but tenuous. Theoretically, BPT may be an early onset variant of basilar migraine or a variant of BPV. Additionally, there is often a family history of migraine.

The differential diagnosis must include gastroesophageal reflux (Sandifer's syndrome), idiopathic torsional dystonia, and complex partial seizure, but particular attention must be paid to the posterior fossa and craniocervical junction where congenital or acquired lesions may produce torticollis. Rarely, trochlear nerve dysfunction produces compensatory head tilt.

Cyclic Vomiting Syndrome

Cyclic vomiting syndrome is an enigmatic symptom complex in young infants and children characterized by repeated stereotyped bouts of pernicious vomiting, often to the point of dehydration. Over the past decade, over 60 articles have been contributed to the existing literature on CVS. Diagnostic criteria have been established. The qualitative clinical criteria for CVS require episodic vomiting with interval wellness and a quantitative requirement for high peak intensity of emisis ($\geq$ 4 emeses/hour) and low episode frequency ($\leq$ 2 episodes/week).[52]

The mechanism of CVS is incompletely understood and, to quote Li in a recent editorial, there may well be "a complex pathophysiologic matrix" underlying CVS.[53] Migraine remains among the possible explanations.

The link between CVS and migraine has traditionally been based on the strong family history of migraine, the episodic nature of CVS, and the shared list of provocative influences including stress and excitement. Further support has been presented recently with autonomic neurocardiac data, which show a commonality of sympathetic nervous system alterations between CVS and migraine.[54] The link has been further strengthened by the favorable clinical response of CVS patients to migraine prophylactic agents cyproheptadine and amitriptyline, with decreased frequency and severity of attacks.[55]

Li et al. examined the overlap between CVS and migraine in a population of 214 children who have CVS and found that 82% had migraine-associated CVS based on either a positive family history or the subsequent development of typical migraine attacks. The authors support a continuum wherein migraine presents with different patterns at various ages: cyclic vomiting in toddlers, abdominal migraine in school-aged children, and migraine headache in older children.[56]

Before this clinical entity can be comfortably diagnosed, cautious and thorough investigations for gastrointestinal disturbances or obstruction (e.g., duplications, stenosis, intussusception), intracranial hypertension (e.g., diencephalic tumors, subdural effusions, hydrocephalus), and inborn errors of metabolism, particularly urea cycle defects and organic acidemias, must be sought.

Li et al. reported a series of 225 children less than 18 years of age who had experienced at least three episodes of vomiting before presenting to their gastroenterology clinic at Columbus Children's Hospital. Between attacks, these children were healthy. Eighty-eight percent were diagnosed as idiopathic CVS but only after extensive negative evaluation. Critically, 41% had associated comorbid disorders that were felt to be contributors to the vomiting. Their excellent study emphasized the point that CVS is not a single diagnostic entity but rather a clinical presentation that can result from "heterogenous disorders."[57]

The treatment of CVS is empiric and parallels that of migraine with the prudent use of prophylactic medications and intensive use of antiemetics plus hydration during attacks. Fleisher's recent editorial outlines a rational course of treatment beyond the scope of this chapter.[58]

Abdominal Migraine

Abdominal migraine is a poorly understood and even more poorly characterized phenomenon of childhood. It presents with repeated stereotyped bouts of unexplained abdominal pain and nausea and vomiting in childhood. The diagnosis is entertained after exhaustive gastrointestinal and metabolic evaluations have been unrevealing. One may cautiously propose that abdominal migraine may be a variant of CVS. As with the preceding variants, headache is infrequently described, except perhaps, in the course of long-term follow-up.

Since abdominal pain is one of the key features of childhood migraine, few would argue that a small subset of children with recurrent, unexplained abdominal pain may represent a spectrum of childhood migraine.

Management

The management of recurrent episodes of the migraine variants is similar to that of migraine with or without aura and incorporates confident reassurance as to the absence of serious underlying disease, general life-style measures, plus a tailored selection of analgesic, antiemetic, and/or prophylactic agents.[59]

The acute treatment of the migraine variants has been the source of much debate, speculation, and myth. The essential issue stems from the concern that some degree of vasoconstriction and hypoperfusion underlies the focal findings. Since many of the available agents for the acute treatment of migraine attacks have strong vasoconstrictive qualities, the logical concern is that localized oligemia may be aggravated and tissue ischemia may result with their use. There are, however, no published reports of cerebrovascular infarction associated with the use of ergotamines or the 5-hydroxytryptamine (5-HT) agonists in migraine variants in children or adolescents. There are no practice parameters or guidelines on the subject. Furthermore, the overwhelming majority of clinical trials assessing the efficacy of 5-HT agonists in children specifically exclude migraine variants from enrollment, so it is unlikely that any data, other than anecdotal reports, will be available in the foreseeable future. Each physician must make this decision carefully on a case-by-case basis, weighing these theoretic risks. No conclusion can be drawn at this time.

Alternative choices of analgesics would include the usual agents such as acetaminophen, ibuprofen, naproxen, or ketorolac tromethamine, coupled with an antiemetic (see Chapter 6, "Pharmacologic Treatment of Headache").

Those patients with frequent or disabling attacks may be considered for daily prophylaxis. Unfortunately, there is a paucity of controlled data published on the prophylactic treatment of the common forms of migraine, and there have been no clinical trial data reported focusing on the prevention of migraine variants. Current common practice is to use those agents addressed in Chapter 6. For those patients with "stroke-like" attacks, there may be some argument for the use of daily doses of baby aspirin, which must be stopped during febrile illness because of concerns of Reye's syndrome.

OTHER PRIMARY HEADACHE SYNDROMES

Tension-Type Headache

Tension-type headache may be hard to differentiate from migraine in children as some of the symptoms overlap. A characteristic tension-type headache is identified by a bilateral pressing tightness occurring anywhere on the cranium or suboccipital region. The headache is nonthrobbing and of mild to moderate intensity and lasts from 30 minutes to several days. It is not accompanied by nausea or vomiting, and it is not aggravated by routine physical activity, although it can be associated with either photophobia or phonophobia (Table 5–10). Rather than using traditional terms, such as muscle contraction headache, tension headache, or stress headache, a new IHS classification employs the term "tension-type" and gives it a rather complex definition for more accurate description.[1] Chronic tension-type headache/chronic daily headache is addressed in Chapter 7.

Cluster Headache

Although cluster headache is very rare under the age of 10 years, it has been reported in children as young as 3 years.[60] Therefore, it should be included

Table 5–10   Episodic Tension-Type Headache (IHS 2.1): Diagnostic Criteria

A. At least 10 previous headache episodes

B. Headache lasting from 30 minutes to 7 days

C. At least two of the following:

 1. Pressing/tightening (nonpulsating) quality

 2. Mild or moderate intensity

 3. Bilateral location

 4. No aggravation by walking stairs or similar routine physical activity

D. Both of the following:

 1. No nausea or vomiting

 2. Photophobia and phonophobia are absent, or one but not the other is present

Adapted from: Classification and diagnostic criteria for headache disorders, cranial neuralgias and facial pain. Headache Classification Committee of the International Headache Society. Cephalalgia 1988;8(Suppl 7):1–96.

Table 5–11   Cluster Headache (IHS 3.1): Diagnostic Criteria

A. At least five attacks fulfilling B and C
B. Severe unilateral orbital, supraorbital, and/or temporal pain lasting 15–180 minutes untreated
C. Headache associated with at least one of the following signs that have to be present on the pain side:
   1. Conjunctival injection
   2. Lacrimation
   3. Nasal congestion
   4. Rhinorrhea
   5. Forehead and facial sweating
   6. Miosis
   7. Ptosis
   8. Eyelid edema

Adapted from: Classification and diagnostic criteria for headache disorders, cranial neuralgias and facial pain. Headache Classification Committee of the International Headache Society. Cephalalgia 1988;8(Suppl 7):1–96.

among the differential diagnoses of primary headaches, although not at the top of the list. Cluster headache becomes more apparent between the ages of 10 and 20 years, and from 20 we see the usual rate of 9 males to 1 female (Table 5–11). For further discussion on cluster headache, see Chapter 10.

CONCLUSION

Migraine headaches affect a gradually increasing proportion of children, from about 1.5% in early childhood to as many as 20% of adolescent females. The majority of affected children will have migraine without aura manifest as recurrent frontal or unilateral nauseating pounding headaches. Migraine variants may present with dramatic neurologic signs, such as ataxia, vertigo, hemiparesis, ophthalmoparesis, or acute confusional states, and must be considered diagnoses of exclusion. Careful anatomic, electrographic, metabolic, toxicologic, and hematologic investigations are usually needed to exclude more ominous underlying disorders.

REFERENCES

1. Classification and diagnostic criteria for headache disorders, cranial neuralgias and facial pain. Headache Classification Committee of the International Headache Society. Cephalalgia 1988;8(Suppl 7):1–96.

2. Gladstein J, Holden EW, Peralta L, Raven M. Diagnoses and symptom patterns in children presenting to a pediatric headache clinic. Headache 1993;33:497–500.

3. Congdon PS, Forsythe WI. Migraine in childhood: a study of 300 children. Dev Med Child Neurol 1979;21:209–216.

4. Seshia SS, Wolstein JR, Adams C, Booth PA, Regin JD, International Headache Society criteria and childhood headache. Dev Med Child Neurol 1994;36: 419–428.

5. Valquist B. Migraine in children. Int Arch Allergy Immunol 1955;7:348–355.

6. Vahlquist B, Hackzell G. Migraine of early onset: a study of 31 cases in which the disease first appeared between 1 and 4 years of age. Acta Paediatr 1949;38:622–636.

7. Bille B. Migraine in school children. Acta Paediatr 1962;51(Suppl 136):1–151.

8. Prensky AL. Migraine and migrainous variants in pediatric patients. Pediatr Clin North Am 1976;23:461–471.

9. Prensky AL, Sommer D. Diagnosis and treatment of migraine in children. Neurology 1979;29:506–510.

10. Milichap JG. Recurrent headaches in 100 children. Electroencephalic abnormalities and response to phenytoin. Child Brain 1978;4:95–104.

11. Passchier J, Bonke B. Migraine symptoms in school children: what is the best diagnostic characteristic for migraine? Headache 1985;25:416–420.

12. Sillanpaa M. Changes in the prevalence of migraine and other headaches during the first seven school years. Headache 1983;23:15–19.

13. Winner P, Wasiewski W, Gladstein J, Linder S. Multicenter prospective evaluation of proposed pediatric migraine revisions to the IHS criteria. Pediatric Headache Committee of the American Association for the Study of Headache. Headache 1997;37:545–548.

14. Winner P, Martinez W, Mate L, Bello L. Classification of pediatric migraine: proposed revisions of the IHS criteria. Headache 1995;35:407–410.

15. Winner P. Headaches in children. Postgrad Med J 1997;101(5):81–90.

16. Winner P, Putnam G, Saiers J, et al. Demographic and migraine characteristics of adolescents clinical trails database. Presented at Headache World 2000, London, UK, September, 2000.

17. Rothner AD. Headaches in children: a review, Headache 1979:19:156–161.

18. Rothner AD. Classification, pathogenesis, evaluation and management of headaches in children and adolescents. Curr Opin Pediatr 1992:4:949–956.

19. Elser JM, Woody RC. Migraine in the infant and young child. Headache 1990;30:366.

20. Hachinski VC, Porchawka J, Steele JC. Visual symptoms in the migraine syndrome. Neurology 1973;23:570–579.

21. Swaiman KF, Frank Y. Seizure headache in children. Dev Med Child Neurol 1978;20:580.

22. Young GB, Blume WT. Painful epileptic seizures. Brain 1983;106:537.

23. Barlow CF. Headaches and migraine in childhood. Clin Dev Med 1984;91: 93–103.

24. Joutel A, Bousser M-G, Biousse V, et al. A gene for familial hemiplegic migraine maps to chromosome 19. Nat Genet 1993;5:40–45.

25. Ophoff RA, Terwindt GM, Vergouwe MN, et al. Wolff-Award 1997. Involvement of a Ca2+ channel gene in familial hemiplegic migraine and migraine with and without aura. Dutch Migraine Genetics Research Group. Headache 1997;37:479–485.

26. Gardner K, Barmada MM, Ptacek LJ, et al. A new locus for hemiplegic migraine maps to chromosome 1q31. Neurology 1997;49:1231–1238.

27. Verret S, Steele JC. Alternating hemiplegia in childhood: a report of eight patients with complicated migraine beginning in infancy. Pediatrics 1971;47:675–680.

28. Aicardi J, Bourgeois M, Goutieres F. Alternating hemiplegia of childhood: clinical findings and diagnostic criteria. In: Andermann F, Aicardi J, Vigevano F, eds. Alternating Hemiplegia of Childhood. New York: Raven Press, 1995, pp 3–18.

29. Rho JM, Chugani HT. Alternating hemiplegia of childhood: insights into its pathogenesis. J Child Neurol 1998;13:39–45.

30. Bickerstaff ER. Basilar artery migraine. Lancet 1961;1:15–17.

31. Lapkin ML, Golden GS. Basilar artery migraine. A review of 30 cases. Am J Dis Child 1978;132:278–281.

32. Barlow CF. Headaches and migraine in childhood. Clin Dev Med 1984;91: 103–109.

33. Golden GS, French JH. Basilar artery migraine in young children. Pediatrics 1975;56:722–726.

34. La Spina I, Vignati A, Porazzi D. Basilar artery migraine: transcranial Doppler EEG and SPECT from the aura phase to the end. Headache 1997;37:43–47.

35. Hansen SL, Borelli-Moller L, Strange P, et al. Ophthalmoplegic migraine: diagnostic criteria, incidence of hospitalization and possible etiology. Acta Neurol Scand 1990;81:54–60.

36. Woody RC, Blaw ME. Ophthalmoplegic migraine in infancy. Clin Pediatr (Phila) 1986;25:82–84.

37. Vijayan N. Ophthalmoplegic migraine: ischemic or compressive neuropathy? Headache 1980;20:300–304.

38. Stommel EW, Ward TN, Harris RD. Ophthalmoplegic migraine or Tolosa–Hunt syndrome? Headache 1994;34:177.

39. Mark AS, Casselman J, Brown D, et al. Ophthalmoplegic migraine; reversible enhancement and thickening of the cisternal segment of the oculomotor nerve on contrast–enhanced MR images. AJNR Am J Neuroradiol 1998;19:1887–1891.

40. May A, Shepheard SL, Knorr M, et al. Retinal plasma extravasation in animals but not in humans: implications for the pathophysiology of migraine. Brain 1998;121:1231–1237.

41. Gascon G, Barlow CF. Juvenile migraine, presenting as acute confusional states. Pediatrics 1970;45:628–635.

42. Ehyai A, Fenichel G. The natural history of acute confusional migraine. Arch Neurol 1978;35:368–369.

43. Jensen TS. Transient global amnesia in childhood. Dev Med Child Neurol 1980;22:654–658.

44. Ferrera PC, Reicho PR. Acute confusional migraine and trauma-triggered migraine. Am J Emerg Med 1996;14:276–278.

45. Amit R. Acute confusional state in childhood. Childs Nerv Syst 1988;4:255–258.

46. Fenichel GM. Migraine as a cause of benign paroxysmal vertigo of childhood. J Pediatr 1967;71:114–115.

47. Basser LS. Benign paroxysmal vertigo of childhood. Brain 1964;87:141.

48. Lanzi G, Balottin U, Fazzi E, et al. Benign paroxysmal vertigo of childhood: a long-term follow-up. Cephalalgia 1994;14:458–460.

49. Chaves-Carballo E. Paroxysmal torticollis. Semin Pediatr Neurol 1996;3: 255–256.

50. Chutorian AM. Benign paroxysmal torticollis, tortipelvis and retrocollis of infancy. Neurology 1974;24:366–367.

51. Snyder CH. Paroxysmal torticollis in infancy. A possible form of labyrinthitis. Am J Dis Child 1969;117:458–460.

52. Pfau BT, Li BUK, Murray RD, et al. Differentiating cyclic vomiting from chronic vomiting patterns in children: quantitative criteria and diagnostic implications. Pediatrics 1996;97:364–368.

53. Li BUK. Cyclic vomiting syndrome: light emerging from the black box. J Pediatr 1999;135:276–277.

54. To J, Issenman RM, Kamath MV. Evaluation of neurocardiac signals in pediatric patients with cyclic vomiting syndrome through power spectral

analysis of heart rate variability. J Pediatr 1999;135:363–366.

55. Andersen JM, Sugerman KS, Lockhart JR, et al. Effective prophylactic therapy for cyclic vomiting syndrome in children using amitriptyline and cyproheptadine. Pediatric 1997;100:977–981.

56. Li BUK, Murray RD, Heitlinger LA, et al. Is cyclic vomiting syndrome related to migraine? J Pediatr 1999;134:567–572.

57. Li BUK, Murray RD, Heitlinger LA, et al. Heterogeneity of diagnoses presenting as cyclic vomiting. Pediatrics 1998;102:583–587.

58. Fleisher DR. Cyclic vomiting syndrome and migraine. J Pediatr 1999;134: 533–535.

59. Lewis DW. Migraine and migraine variant in childhood and adolescence. Semin Pediatr Neurol 1995;2:127–143.

60. Kudrow L. Cluster Headache: Mechanisms and Management. Oxford, England: Oxford University Press, 1980.

Chapter 6

PHARMACOLOGIC TREATMENT OF HEADACHE

Paul Winner, Steven L. Linder,
and Warren W. Wasiewski

Recent advances in the management of headache for adults have translated into improved treatment for children and adolescents. Recent studies conducted in children and adolescents are helping us to outline appropriate management strategies for this population. The potential to control pediatric migraine in 1 to 2 hours has now been documented.

The diagnosis of a benign (primary) headache needs to satisfy the patient, parent, and practitioner. Practitioners should take this opportunity to review the causative mechanisms with both the patient and the parents, as well as provide a comprehensive treatment approach including both pharmacologic and nonpharmacologic methods, as appropriate for the individual patient. The majority of childhood headache patients who are brought to a physician for evaluation will prove to have a diagnosis of migraine.[1,2] To effectively treat sick episodic headache (migraine), the physician initially needs to identify potential triggers and outline an acute treatment strategy with a goal of eliminating headache pain in 1 to 2 hours. If the initial medication is not fully effective, the physician needs to consider either repeating the initial medication or starting a possible rescue medication with the goal of eliminating all pain symptoms by 4 hours. In this age group, especially children under the age of 12 years, headache may last only 1 to 2 hours. In this case, a more moderate approach toward treatment and pain relief can be used.[3–6] When appropriate, preventive treatment strategies should be designed with a goal of reducing headache frequency by approximately 50%, with a possible reduction of headache severity. Moreover, they should be used on average for 6-month periods, with re-evaluation. Since there is a relatively high remission rate of migraine in children, it is often possible to taper a preventive regimen within 6 months of its initiation.

ACUTE TREATMENT STRATEGIES

Parents and their children want an effective and safe method of removal of headache pain, as well as a lessening of the disability. For children and adolescents with mild to moderate migraine, mild analgesics, combination analgesics, and nonsteroidal anti-inflammatory drugs (NSAIDs) are often quite effective (Table 6–1). It is important in young children and adolescents to discuss the issue of rebound headache in an effort to avoid its occurrence. Butalbital-containing compounds and mild analgesics can be used safely and effectively in young children and adolescents, but some limits need to be provided. At the Palm Beach Headache Center, we suggest no more than 10 tablets of an analgesic per month for a young child and no more than 20 tablets for an adolescent, with no more than 2 to 3 headaches treated with these parameters per week. With the assistance of a parent and a diary, these parameters can be followed rather easily.

In a recent study of childhood headache at school entry, it was noted that 24% of children had seen a doctor for their headache complaints. The medications that were taken were ibuprofen (36%), acetaminophen (30%), salicylic acid (27%), and naproxen (8%); it was noted that 47% of these children received medication for every headache.[7] The Food and

Table 6–1   Acute Treatment

Simple Analgesics	Dosage
Acetaminophen	10–15 mg/kg
Ibuprofen	10 mg/kg
Naproxen sodium	10 mg/kg
Combination Analgesic	
Fioricet®	Butalbital 50 mg, acetaminophen 325 mg, caffeine 40 mg
Esgic*plus*®	Butalbital 50 mg, acetaminophen 500 mg, caffeine 40 mg
Axocet®	Butalbital 50 mg, acetaminophen 500 mg

Drug Administration (FDA) approves the use of ibuprofen and naproxen for use in children over the age of 2 years. Although Reye's syndrome is rare, salicylates should be avoided in children who are febrile and/or in whom there is concern for an underlying metabolic disorder.

Triptans

Children, like adults, want relief for their symptoms as quickly as possible (Table 6–2). The introduction of the 5-hydroxytryptamine (5-HT$_1$) agonists has revolutionized the treatment of children with moderate to severe migraine. The 5-HT$_1$ agonists are now being studied in adolescents so that they too may benefit from this form of therapy when appropriate. Linder, in an open-label study,[8] documented the effectiveness of subcutaneous sumatriptan 0.06 mg per kg and showed an overall efficacy of 72% at 30 minutes and 78% at 2 hours, with a recurrence rate of 6%. Because children tend to have a shorter duration of headache, a recurrence rate of 6% would seem appropriate for this study population.

Children who prefer to avoid the parenteral route of administration now have the option of using the oral and nasal spray forms of 5-HT$_1$ agonists.[6] Sumatriptan has been studied in a double-blind, placebo-controlled trial of 25-, 50-, and 100-mg tablets in 302 adolescents in 35 sites.[9] Sumatriptan was statistically significant over the placebo at 25, 50, and 100 mg at the 180- and 240-minute mark showing 74% pain relief at the 4-hour mark. The primary end point of the study was at 2 hours, and statistical significance was not met due to a high placebo rate, which in this adolescent study may be due in part to study design. If adult placebo rates are substituted at the 2-hour mark, statistical significance would be obtained. New study designs are being implemented to address the special issues of the pediatric population; for example, the fact that children have a shorter

Table 6–2   Acute Treatment of Moderate to Severe Migraine

5-HT$_1$ agonists (triptan)

Ergotamine (dihydroergotamine)

Nonsteroidal anti-inflammatory drugs

Antiemetics

Opioid analgesic

duration of headache. The headache recurrence rates varied from 18 to 28% across all three doses[9] and were lower than those seen in adults possibly because children tend to have a shorter duration of headache. No significant adverse events were documented in this study of 302 patients.[9] The side effects of the placebo and 25 mg of sumatriptan were almost identical. As the dose was increased to 50 mg, there was a slight increase in side effects reported, and then a further increase reported at 100 mg. For example, the 50-mg dose side effects of a feeling of warmth, tightness, burning, stinging, numbness, strangeness, and pressure ranged from 1 to 4%. This compared with the range of 0 to 1% at the 25-mg tablet dose. The side effects of chest discomfort, tightness, pressure and heaviness ranged from 0 to 1% for the 25-mg tablets as compared with 0 to 3% for the placebo and 3 to 4% for the 50-mg tablets. Cardiovascular palpitations, tachyarrhythmias, and hypotension were reported to be 0 to 1% for the 25- and 50-mg tablets and slightly higher for the 100-mg tablets. No such side effects were reported in the placebo group. The study demonstrated that 25-, 50-, and 100-mg oral tablets of sumatriptan were effective in treating acute migraine, with similar efficacy profiles across all three dosages.

Adolescents should begin with 25-mg sumatriptan tablets for the treatment of migraine. If they do not have complete relief within 2 hours, the dose should be repeated. Should 25 mg not be effective, the dose needs to be increased to 50 mg as the initial dose and repeated in 2 hours, if needed. Rescue medication can be used at anytime for the relief of associated symptoms, but often with triptans it is not necessary. The goal, much like in adults, is to obtain a pain-free status for the child or adolescent at 2 hours; if this has not occurred, the same triptan medication needs to be repeated so that the patient is pain-free by 4 hours. Although the associated symptoms of migraine such as nausea, photophobia, or phonophobia often respond to tripan, they may not be completely relieved.

Sumatriptan nasal spray was studied in a randomized, double-blind, placebo-controlled trial in which adolescents ages 12 to 17 years were treated for a single attack[10] with three nasal spray doses: 5, 10, and 20 mg. At 1 hour, 56% of patients using the 10- or 20-mg dose of sumatriptan nasal spray reported significant postdose headache relief compared with 41% in the placebo group.[10] All three doses were superior to the placebo with respect to the cumulative percentage of patients who obtained headache relief within 2 hours of administration; 66% of adolescents receiving the 5-mg dose reported headache relief that was statistically superior as compared with the placebo. When reviewing the pain-free data, the 20-mg sumatriptan nasal spray provided a statistically significant greater response of 36% at 2 hours postdose compared with the placebo at 25% ($p < .05$).[10] It should be noted that each dose of sumatriptan was superior to the placebo with respect to the cumulative percentage of patients reporting pain-free response 2 hours postdose. When looking at the associated symptoms, photophobia was significantly lower with the 20-mg sumatriptan nasal spray at 2 hours compared with the placebo.

There were no differences noted in the rescue medication of the second dose of sumatriptan in either the sumatriptan or placebo groups. Also, there was no difference in headache recurrence among the treatment groups, which ranged from 16 to 20%, and the placebo group at 20%. Again, note that the recurrence rates tend to be lower in adolescent groups than in adult groups, possibly due to the shorter duration of headaches in the adolescent population. Headache recurrence was lower in the 10- and 20-mg sumatriptan nasal spray patient groups at 8 hours and 8.2 hours respectively as compared with the placebo group at 6.7 hours (Table 6–3).[10]

The most common adverse event reported by this patient group was taste disturbance. If this is removed from the calculations, the overall incidence of adverse events for the nasal treatment group is similar to the placebo group. No serious adverse event was reported in the sumatriptan treatment population in this study. Overall, 20-mg sumatriptan nasal spray provided the most rapid treatment across this adolescent population group. It also proved to be well tolerated, and the results are similar to those reported in the adult sumatriptan nasal spray clinical trials.[11–13]

Table 6–3   Triptans for Acute Treatment in Adolescents

Triptan	Form	Dose
Sumatriptan (Imitrex)	Subcutaneous	0.06 mg/kg up to 6 mg
	Nasal spray	5 mg, 20 mg
	Tablet	25 mg, 50 mg
Rizatriptan (Maxalt)	Tablet	5 mg
(Maxalt MLT)	Orally disintegrating tablet	5 mg
Zolmitriptan (Zomig)	Tablet	2.5 mg, 5 mg

The disturbance in taste can be reduced by the use of flavored lozenges or hard candy (lemon drops) after administration of the nasal spray. Despite the reported taste disturbance by some patients, this does not discourage adolescents from the continued use of the nasal spray medication.[14] The taste disturbance also may be lessened by re-instructing adolescents in the correct administration of the nasal spray medication.[10]

Rizatriptan (Maxalt) 5-mg tablets have been recently evaluated in patients ages 12 to 17 years in a double-blind, placebo-controlled, parallel-group, single-attack study. A total of 149 adolescents were treated with rizatriptan 5 mg, and 147 were treated with a placebo. The majority of patients used one dose of study medication. The percentage of adolescents receiving pain relief at 2 hours for the rizatriptan 5-mg group was 66%; this is similar to that seen in the adult population receiving a 5-mg dose but is not statistically significant since the response of the placebo group was 57%. The headache-free status at 2 hours was 32% for the rizatriptan 5-mg group and 28% for the placebo. There were no serious adverse events in the adolescent patient rizatriptan population. The most common adverse events reported were fatigue, dizziness, somnolence, dry mouth, and nausea. With regard to functional disability, significantly more adolescent patients (44%) on rizatriptan 5 mg had no functional disability at 2 hours as compared with the placebo group (36%). Rizatriptan 5 mg is well tolerated in this adolescent population study.[15]

Zolmitriptan (Zomig) has been studied in a subgroup of adolescents (12 to 17 years). The first two migraine subgroups were treated with 2.5 mg and subsequent attacks with 2.5 or 5 mg at each patient's discretion. The overall headache response at 2 hours was 80% (88% and 70% with zolmitriptan, 2.5 mg and 5 mg respectively). Treatment was well tolerated.[16] Further double-blind, placebo-controlled studies of triptans are in progress, including rizatriptan (Maxalt), zolmitriptan (Zomig), naratriptan (Amerge), and eletriptan, which are under various stages of evaluation regarding the pediatric and adolescent population.

Ergot Alkaloids

The ergot alkaloids are a family of chemicals that have many pharmacologic effects. Their diversity results from their interaction with multiple receptors, their variable receptor affinity and intrinsic activity, and their variable organ-specific receptor access. Ergotamine tartrate (ET) was one of the first ergot alkaloids to be isolated. Dihydroergotamine (DHE) (tradename D.H.E. 45) is a synthetic ergot with a modified pharmacologic profile. Both ET and DHE have $5\text{-}HT_{1A}$–, $5\text{-}HT_{1B}$–, $5\text{-}HT_{1D}$–, and $5\text{-}HT_{1F}$–receptor agonist affinity. Dihydroergotamine exhibits a greater α-adrenergic antagonist activity and has less potent arterial vasoconstriction and emetic potential than ET. Dihydroergotamine was first reported to be effective in migraine by Horton et al. in 1945.[17] Unfortunately, the medication fell into disuse until Raskin reintroduced it in 1986.[18]

Dihydroergotamine offers numerous benefits compared with ET because of a lower reported incidence of nausea and vomiting, as well as a lower headache recurrence and lack of rebound headache. Intravenous administration in adults provides an effective form of rapid headache relief for migraine and often is used for refractory severe migraine headache patients. Linder has studied the use of DHE in children and adolescents. Rapid administration of intravenous DHE in children can be associated with adverse events and a more constant rate of infusion is recommended with a coadministered antiemetic, for example promethazine hydrochloride or metoclopramide hydrochloride.

In adults, the oral form of DHE is poorly absorbed and ineffective for acute migraine. Intramuscular or subcutaneous administration can be effective for moderate to severe migraine.[19] Intranasal delivery vehicles also have been shown to be effective in adults. However, no studies involving intramuscular, nasal, or oral forms of DHE in children or adolescents have been done. Limited work using intravenous forms has been performed.[19,20]

Articles have been published outlining the use of DHE in adolescents and children in both inpatient and outpatient settings.[20,21] Prior to initiating an outpatient protocol (Table 6–4) or an inpatient protocol (Table 6–5), a

Table 6–4   Dihydroergotamine Protocol: Outpatient Treatment

Age (Years)	Metoclopramide (Per Dose)*	Dihydroergotamine (Per Dose)†
6–9	0.2 mg/kg	0.1 mg
9–12	0.2 mg/kg	0.2 mg
12–16	0.2 mg/kg	0.25 mg

*Metoclopramide is administered orally 30 minutes prior to the administration of intravenous dihydroergotamine. The maximum dose is 15 mg.
†Dihydroergotamine is diluted with 30–60 cc normal saline and given over 30–60 minutes.

detailed history and physical and neurologic examinations are necessary to clinically define the situation. Girls must be evaluated appropriately for concerns of pregnancy when necessary. Neuroimaging studies may be necessary if there is concern about the intracranial pathology. However, this normally can be excluded by a thorough history and physical examination. In patients who have a prolonged migraine and especially atypical migraine, laboratory studies may be helpful to exclude other related medical problems.

Although reports of serious adverse events on recommended doses of DHE are rare, side effects can be seen with either the antiemetic metoclopramide or DHE (Table 6–6). In children and adolescents, the dosing of DHE is extremely important for both efficacy and the prevention of adverse events. Dihydroergotamine, which often needs dose adjustment depending on the patient's age, can be used in an intravenous form concomitantly with an antiemetic: ages 6 to 9 years, 0.1 mg per dose; ages 9 to 12 years, 0.2 mg per dose; and ages 12 to 16 years, 0.3 to 0.5 mg per dose.[20] The intramuscular and subcutaneous forms can be used without a concomitant antiemetic. The initial dose of DHE is recommended to be given in the emergency department or office at the onset of a migraine headache, and if there is incomplete relief of the headache symptoms within 1 hour, a second dose may be given.

Table 6–5   Dihydroergotamine Protocol: Inpatient Treatment*

Age (Years)	Antiemetic (PO) (Per Dose)†	Dihydroergotamine (IV) (Per Dose)‡
6–9	Metoclopramide 0.2mg/kg	0.1 mg
9–12	Metoclopramide 0.2 mg/kg	0.15 mg
12–16	Metoclopramide 0.2 mg/kg	0.2 mg

PO = per os (by mouth); IV = intravenous.
*For prolonged vascular headache, PO metoclopramide and IV dihydroergotamine (DHE) should be repeated every 6 hours for a maximum of 12 doses. When the headache ceases, an additional dose should be given.
†The antiemetic should be administered PO, to a maxium dose of 15 mg, 30 minutes prior to the IV DHE. If extrapyramidal syndrome develops, diphenhydramine hydrochloride, 1 mg/kg (maximum dose of 50 mg), should be given and metoclopramide discontinued. For subsequent treatments, ondansetron hydrochloride, 0.15 mg/kg IV or PO, should be administered 30 minutes prior to the appropriate DHE dose.
‡The DHE may be increased by 0.05 mg/dose to the point where the patient has mild abdominal discomfort. The protocol should be continued at the dose prior to the onset of the abdominal discomfort. If a significant myofascial component develops, then IV ketorolac tromethamine 7.5–15 mg/6 h should be used alternating with DHE.

Dihydroergotamine is a medication that often requires dosage titration.[20] For example, one of the more common side effects, nausea, actually may indicate that the dose is slightly high. It may be helpful to give adolescents or children a test dose of DHE on a day when they do not have a migraine to determine if the treatment causes any significant nausea. In general, side effects can be avoided by lowering the dose or by diluting the DHE with 30 to 60 cc of saline and administering it over a period of 30 minutes to 1 hour intravenously.[20] In addition, 20 to 30 minutes prior to the administration of DHE, metoclopramide should be given to prevent nausea or vomiting.[20] In addition to preventing nausea, metoclopramide has antidopaminergic effects and thus may also be helpful in treating migraine. Note that pediatric patients are extremely sensitive to some antiemetics, including metoclopramide, and may develop extrapyramidal side effects. This is especially true when the medication is given in an intravenous form. These extrapyramidal side effects are readily reversed using diphenhydramine at a dose of 1 mg per kg up to 50 mg. The extrapyramidal side effects can also be seen using the oral form of metoclopramide, and if this is the case, it is normally seen between the fifth and eighth dose, and, again, is readily reversible with diphenhydramine. If the patient has difficulty with metoclopramide, promethazine hydrochloride may be substituted. Dihydroergotamine has been used in pediatric patients since the early 1990s as an effective treatment of moderate to severe migraine headaches. Since triptan medications have been approved for the treatment of migraine, DHE is used less frequently, but it still is a reliable alternative should triptans prove to be ineffective or their side effects prove intolerable. Dihydroergotamine also has proven to be useful for migraine headaches that last more than 2 to 4 days (status migrainosus).[22] Both inpatient and outpatient DHE protocols may be used to break intractable migraine headaches. The use of DHE,

Table 6–6   Side Effects

Metoclopramide	Dihydroergotamine
Extrapyramidal dysfunction	Flushed feeling
Akathisia, "itching in head"	Nausea/vomiting
	Tingling in extremities
	Leg cramping
	Transient increase in headache

as well as triptans, is contraindicated in patients with certain high-risk factors such as uncontrolled hypertension, carotid or peripheral artery disease, and thyrotoxicosis. Caution is advised for patients with a history of congenital heart disease or other medical problems (Table 6–7).

Antiemetics

Antiemetics, both the suppository and the oral forms, can be used in children and adolescents with acute migraine accompanied by nausea or vomiting. Promethazine hydrochloride, either the 25- or 50-mg suppository form, can prove to be quite efficacious in the younger child who has significant vomiting associated with migraine; in children who have nausea symptoms without vomiting either the 25- or 50-mg tablet form can be used. Prochlorperazine maleate and metoclopramide can also be quite effective, although they should be used with caution because of potential extrapyramidal side effects. Antiemetics can be used quite effectively in conjunction with other acute therapies for treating moderate to severe migraine in children and adolescents.

Analgesics

In children under the age of 6 years limited amounts of acetaminophen are effective and cause few problems since headaches are short lived and resolve with sleep. In older children acetaminophen, NSAIDs, and butalbital-containing analgesic compounds may be useful in the absence of significant nausea. A brief discussion with patients and parents about the potential of analgesic-induced rebound headache is recommended as a precaution

Table 6–7   Contraindications for the Use of Triptans, Ergot Alkaloids

Symptoms or findings consistent with ischemic heart disease, coronary artery vasospasm, or other significant underlying cardiovascular disease

Uncontrolled hypertension

Hemiplegic or basilar migraine

Use of another 5-HT agonist or ergot-type medication (dihydroergotamine) within 24 hours of treatment

Administration of monoamine oxidase inhibitors within previous 2 weeks

Hypersensitivity to a triptan or any of its inactive ingredients against long-term abuse. In children under the age of 15 years aspirin can be used with caution provided the patient is afebrile and has no suggestion of a metabolic disorder because of the concerns of Reye's syndrome.[23]

Opioids such as meperidine hydrochloride and codeine can be used in children over the age of 6 years with caution and physician supervision.[23]

Case Presentation: A 12-year-old girl presents with a 6-month history of episodic incapacitating headaches. These headaches occur, on average, three to four times a month. They begin gradually in the bifrontal region and intensify over 1 to 2 hours to an incapacitating, throbbing pain that worsens with activity. The girl reports associated nausea and photophobia. The headaches, which last 4 to 12 hours, often are precipitated by skipping meals or eating hot dogs. She denies any visual, motor, or sensory changes. There is no reported lightheadedness or dizziness associated with these episodes. She denies any episodes of meningitis, encephalitis, or head trauma. Her past medical history is unremarkable. Her family history is positive for migraine on the maternal side. She reports missing 2 days of school per month due to these headaches. She has attempted to treat these headaches with over-the-counter medications including ibuprofen, with no significant improvement. Her examination is normal except for some diffuse discomfort in the cervical region. Her blood pressure is 98/68, and her pulse is 68 and regular.

This is a 12-year-old girl with a history consistent with the International Headache Society criteria for migraine without aura. This patient presents with bifrontal headache symptomatology, which is often seen in children, especially in the younger age group. Unilateral headache is seen in roughly 60% of adult migraine patients and to a lesser percent in children. This patient also describes having nausea without vomiting. Children often will experience vomiting early in the headache episode, although this patient did not. Children often report photophobia without phonophobia or the reverse.

This patient has reported having similar episodic sick headaches for 6 months with no prominent change in intensity. The possibility of a prominent central nervous system (CNS) lesion in this patient is unlikely as there has been no significant change in headache frequency or severity. Also, the patient had a normal physical examination and a positive family history of migraine. Physicians should have a high index of suspicion for a CNS lesion in a patient under the age of 12 years who has a headache history of less then 4 months with increasing frequency and/or severity, an abnormal physical examination, and no family history of migraine.

This patient was unsuccessful in controlling her migraine with over-the-counter medications. When patients do not respond satisfactorily to analgesics, they may benefit greatly by the use of triptans (e.g., sumatriptan, rizatriptan, [and possibly zolmitriptan and eletriptan pending study results]). This patient may benefit significantly from the use of sumatriptan (Imitrex), 25-mg tablet or 20-mg nasal spray, which can relieve her headache symptoms within 1 to 2 hours. Should the initial triptan not be successful in relieving the headache after at least 2 to 3 headache episodes treated, another triptan at appropriate dosages should be used (see Table 6–3).

This individual has three to four migraines without aura per month. Should this patient continue to not respond to abortive therapy, preventive therapy may be considered.

PREVENTIVE THERAPY STRATEGIES

For those children who do not respond completely to acute treatment of migraine or who are missing excessive amounts of school or have significant interference in there life due to frequent and incapacitating migraine headaches, preventive therapy should be considered. Age can play a role in the selection of appropriate therapy, and often doses need to be tailored to the individual child and adolescent. The preventive therapy of migraine includes not only the pharmacologic treatment but also the identification of migraine triggers, which may involve adjusting lifestyle when appropriate. To date, there are no well-controlled clinical trials with sufficient patient numbers to support the use of any particular agent in the preventive treatment of migraine headaches in children or adolescents. Pertinent literature on the preventive treatment of migraine in children and adolescents, as well as dosing guidelines based on the limited data available and the clinical experience, will be reviewed.

Several issues must be addressed prior to considering the use of a pharmacologic agent. These include an accurate assessment of headache frequency and severity, the effectiveness of current episodic medications, the identification of possible triggers, and most importantly, the degree of disability caused by the headache.

Headache Calendars

Headache calendars are extremely valuable for determining accurate headache frequency, severity, and disability. They can demonstrate patterns of headache occurrence that may not be otherwise apparent. Triggers can be identified if the appropriate information is recorded. Table 6–8 is a

Table 6–8   Migraine Calendar

Date
Time of onset
Any warning symptoms
Pain — scale (0–5)
Rating
Type
Location
Other symptoms
Treatment
Time
Medication
Dose
2 hours later/2nd treatment
Symptoms
Pain
Rating
Type
Location
Treatment
4 hours later/3rd treatment
Symptoms
Pain
Rating
Type
Location
Treatment
Did the headache interfere with activities?

migraine event calendar. Pertinent information recorded on the calendar includes time of onset of the headache; the occurrence of any aura symptoms; and an assessment of the pain intensity, quality, and location. A visual analogue scale may be included, making it easier for the younger patients to use. Associated symptoms, including photophobia, phonophobia, nausea, and vomiting, are also recorded. Patients then record the treatment, noting the time, medication, and dose used. Then they reassess their headache severity 2 hours after the treatment. Headache disability is assessed by determining if the headache interfered with activities. This information is invaluable in assessing the child's headache severity and can help identify specific triggers. In addition, the calendar allows questions to be asked concerning a specific headache event; for example, "What were the child's activities the day before the headache occurred?" For many children, sleep deprivation is a significant trigger and attendance at sleepovers may precipitate a significant headache the following day. When completed, either by the parent or the child, the calendar gives an accurate picture of the child's headache history. With this information in hand, decisions concerning the use of preventive medications or adjustments in acute therapy can be made.

Acute Therapy

In many circumstances, inappropriately low doses of analgesics have been used to treat migraines in children. In addition, it is not uncommon for parents to call and indicate that the child has had a headache for greater than 2 days and only a single dose of medication has been used. There appears to be a significant medication-phobia on the part of the parents who then administer inappropriately low doses of analgesics. With appropriate education and a treatment plan for each headache, this fear can be significantly reduced. In many patients, an appropriate dose of an acute medication at the onset of the headache can be quite effective in reducing the headache's severity or in relieving the headache. Therefore, at the initial evaluation, preventive medications generally should not be started. Patients are requested to track their headache frequency on a calendar as well as follow a specific headache treatment protocol for the next several headaches to determine if appropriate treatment of an acute headache can reduce the headache frequency.

Nonpharmacologic Measures

Nonpharmacologic preventive measures that may reduce headache frequency include sleep hygiene, diet, and exercise. Lack of sleep can be a significant trigger for many children. An alteration of sleep behavior, such as going to bed late or sleeping late, may precipitate headaches. It is quite helpful if the patient arises every morning at the same time. As mentioned earlier, sleepover headaches are quite common. This can be seen even in a patient who has a fairly well-controlled headache disorder.

In addition to sleep hygiene, a regular balanced diet is beneficial. Frequently, adolescents concerned about weight gain may choose not to eat breakfast or lunch. This results in a relatively severe headache later in the day. In the adolescent, both sleep hygiene and diet can be significant triggers that can be somewhat difficult to control.

Although food triggers for migraine headache are relatively infrequent, probably occurring in less than 20% of the patients, identification of such triggers in a particular patient can be quite beneficial.[24] Table 6–9 lists several foods, such as cheese and chocolate, that are known precipitants for headache. The total elimination of these foods from the diet is not necessary; however, it is important for patients to determine if any of those foods are a trigger and if so, attempt to eliminate them from their diet.

Regular physical exercise appears to reduce headache frequency. Although the value of this has never been demonstrated in children, establishing a lifestyle that includes adequate exercise, sleep, and physical activity certainly cannot be harmful to the child's overall well-being.

Stress may play a significant role in precipitating migraine events. Riback identified stress as a provoking factor in 23% of 226 children.[24] As identified in Table 6–9, school and interpersonal relationships are the most significant stresses in the life of an adolescent. Stress management using relaxation techniques and/or biofeedback can be helpful in children who are motivated to use them. Biofeedback has been demonstrated to be effective in children as young as 9 years old (Table 6–10).[25]

When all of the above issues have been addressed, yet the child continues to have disabling headaches at a significant frequency, then a decision to initiate preventive medication needs to be considered. A high frequency of headache alone may not be enough to justify the use of a preventive medication. Headache disability, which can be defined by a variety of headache disability scales but, more importantly, by the impact on the individual patient's life, should be used to determine who should be placed on preventive medication. Certainly, a child experiencing three to four significant migraine headaches a month resulting in disability for several hours each time, deserves to be considered for preventive medication. However, even the child who experiences only one severe headache a month that results in a significant disability (i.e., a headache of 3 days' duration resulting in loss of school time and/or social time) should also be considered for preventive medication.

Table 6–9   Migraine Triggers

Foods
    Ripened cheeses, such as cheddar, Gruyère, Stilton, Brie, and Camembert
    Chocolate
    Vinegars (except white vinegar)
    Sour cream, yogurt
    Nuts, peanut butter
    Hot fresh breads, raised coffeecakes, and doughnuts
    Lima beans, navy beans, and pea pods
    Monosodium glutamate
    Canned figs
    Bananas
    Pizza
    Pork
    Fermented sausages, bologna, pepperoni, hotdogs
    Food dyes
    Sauerkraut
    Caffeine

Odors
    Perfume
    Gasoline
    Various food odors

Stresses
    School work
    Excess number of extracurricular activities
    Relationships: friends, siblings, or parents
    Disruption of lifestyle
    Feeling "bummed out" or sad all the time

Preventive Medications

Although the exact mechanisms of action of the preventive medications studied to date remain largely unproven, they are presumed to act through four main mechanisms: 5-HT$_2$ antagonism, modulation of plasma extravasation, modulation of central aminergic control mechanisms, or membrane stabilizing effects via voltage sensitive channels.[26] Divalproex sodium recently has been shown to be effective in migraine prophylaxis in adults.[27] Divalproex sodium may exert its protective effect by suppressing migraine-related cortical events, perivascular parasympathetic activity, or trigeminal nucleus caudalis activity.[28] Alternatively, it may attenuate nociceptive neurotransmission or suppress neurogenic inflammation. Thus, divalproex sodium may alter migraine genesis at several sites along the pathway, from stimulus to headache pain. Gabapentin, although structurally related to γ-aminobutyric acid (GABA), does not interact with GABA receptors, is not converted to GABA, and is not an inhibitor of GABA uptake or degradation. Thus, gabapentin must exert its effects on migraine genesis through an alternative mechanism other than GABA neurotransmission. Baclofen (Lioresal) is a structural analogue of the inhibitory neurotransmitter GABA and has been reported to be an effective migraine preventive agent. Although its mechanism of action is unknown, it is thought to exert its effects on spasticity by stimulation of GABA(B) receptors.[29] Dotarizine, an experimental 5-HT$_2$ receptor antagonist was recently reported to reduce migraine headache frequency.[30] This is the first report of a designer drug of serotonin antagonism in the preventive treatment of migraine. Thus, there are several potential sites along the pathway of migraine genesis that can be affected by these diverse compounds resulting in migraine prevention.

Table 6–10   Nonpharmacologic Treatment of Migraine

Education

Biofeedback

Stress management and relaxation exercises

Elimination of triggers

Sleep regulation

Exercise

Once the decision to add a pharmacologic agent is made, there are several medications from which to choose. The appropriate dose for any of these agents has not yet been determined. The information provided herein is a summary of the literature, with dosage recommendations based on the few clinical reports as well as clinical experience (Tables 6–11 and 6–12).

Anticonvulsants

Several anticonvulsants have been used for migraine prevention, including phenobarbital, carbamazepine, phenytoin, and divalproex sodium. Intravenous infusion of valproate sodium (Depacon) has recently been reported to abort acute migraine headache.[31] The divalproex sodium migraine prevention study group has shown that 500 to 1500 mg per day of divalproex sodium is effective in reducing headache frequency in adults.[27] Extended-release divalproex sodium (Depakote ER) has been demonstrated to be effective and well tolerated at doses of 500 and 1000 mg once daily in adults.[32] Caruso et al. treated 31 children in the age range of 7 to 16 years with divalproex sodium as a preventive agent.[33] Dosages ranged from 15 to 45 mg per kg per day. After 4 months of treatment, 76% of the patients had a greater than 50% reduction in headache frequency, 18% had a greater than 75% reduction, and 6% were essentially headache-free.[34,35] This study suggests that divalproex sodium may indeed be effective as a migraine preventive agent in children and adolescents.

Clinical experience with divalproex sodium for seizures suggests that 10 mg per kg per day divided twice daily is a safe starting dose (see Table 6–11). The dose can then be increased in the second week of treatment to 15 to 20 mg per kg per day divided either twice or three times a day. There

Table 6–11   Preventive Therapy

Agent	Initial Dosage
Cyproheptadine (Periactin)	2 mg bid or 4 mg hs
Propranolol (Inderal)	1 mg/kg, up to 10 mg bid
Tricyclic antidepressants	
Amitriptyline (Elavil)	0.25–0.5 mg/kg, up to 10 mg hs
Nortriptyline (Pamelor)	0.25–0.5 mg/kg, up to 10 mg hs
Divalproex sodium (Depakote) (sprinkle)	10 mg/kg, up to 125 mg daily

bid = twice daily; hs = at bedtime.

are no data on serum drug levels to suggest a therapeutic range for migraine prevention. The sprinkle formula, 125-mg divalproex capsules, is well tolerated and may help to decrease any potential gastrointestinal side efects. Other reported potential side effects of divalproex sodium include sedation, increased appetite, and temporary hair loss. Divalproex sodium can also reduce platelet counts in a dose-dependent manner; therefore, monitoring of platelet counts should be considered, especially when higher doses are given. Hyperammonemia can also occur from divalproex sodium without elevated transaminases; therefore a serum ammonia level should be obtained from patients who report being excessively tired. Due to the potential teratogenic effects, folic acid, 2 to 4 mg daily, can be added to the treatment for adolescent girls. Divalproex sodium (Depakote) has been approved by the FDA as a treatment for the prevention of migraine (see Table 6–12).

Although the other anticonvulsants have been used by clinicians, there are limited studies to support their use. When used in migraine prevention, the antiepileptic doses are usually prescribed.

Antidepressants

The tricyclic antidepressant amitriptyline has been reported to reduce headache frequency in children.[36,37] However, the efficacy of amitriptyline has not been studied in a placebo-controlled trial. Levinstein compared amitriptyline with propranolol and cyproheptadine in an open-label study.[37] In that study, 30 children were randomized to receive one of the three treatments. It is not noted how many children were treated with amitriptyline. He reports a moderate 50 to 60% improvement to an excellent 80% improvement at 3 months of treatment with amitriptyline. Hershey et al. were more precise in reporting a reduction in headache frequency

Table 6–12   Drugs with FDA Approval for Migraine Prevention

Drug	Year of Approval
Divalproex sodium (Depakote)	1996
Timolol (Blocadren)	1990
Propranolol (Inderal)	1979
Methysergide (Sansert)	1962

FDA = Food and Drug Administration.

in their open-label study but had a mixture of headache types including headaches occurring at a frequency of greater than three per week.[36]

The appropriate dosage of amitriptyline has not yet been determined. Levinstein used a dosage of 15 mg per day.[37] Hershey et al. suggested a standardized dosage of 1 mg per kg per day.[36] This is the first report of standardized dosing of amitriptyline based on body weight.

Clinical experience suggests that a reasonable starting dosage of amitriptyline for a 5- to 10-year-old child is 0.25 to 0.5 mg per kg up to 10 mg per day administered at bedtime (see Table 6–11). For an adolescent, 10 mg is a reasonable starting dose. A dosage ranging from 10 to 75 mg per day is usually effective in reducing headache frequency. Children may experience drowsiness with the medication in the early phases of treatment. This usually resolves over a 2- to 3-week period. In the first 2 to 4 weeks, a 10-mg single daily dosage is usually maintained. At the end of a 2- to 4-week trial, the medication should be titrated upward to either efficacy or intolerable side effects. Because of the potential cardiac side effects, electrocardiography should be performed if dosage escalation is required. A dosage exceeding 75 mg per day is rarely needed to control headache.[22]

Nortriptyline also has been widely used as an alternative to amitriptyline with the belief that there are fewer side effects. The usual starting dosage is 10 mg per day administered at bedtime (see Table 6–11). The side effects of nortriptyline are identical to those of amitriptyline.[23]

Serotonin selective reuptake inhibitors (SSRIs) have been studied in adults but not in children. Fluoxetine has been shown to be effective in treating mild headache in the adult population in a limited study.[38] In our center, the SSRIs are used when there is clinical suspicion of depression. Paroxetine appears to be more efficacious than fluoxetine. A starting dosage of 10 mg per day for the first week increasing to 20 mg per day is suggested. The dosage is usually administered in the morning to avoid difficulties with insomnia. Worsening of headache may occur in some patients. Initially, there is appetite suppression with concomitant weight loss, followed by increased appetite and weight gain. The serotonin syndrome may occur in patients on SSRIs who are treated with 5-HT$_1$ agonists for an acute headache. There are no data to support their use in migraine prevention in children.

Antihistamines

Cyproheptadine, an antihistamine with antiserotoninergic properties, was one of the earliest medications reported to be useful in migraine prevention in children.[39] Although it has antiserotoninergic properties, its antimigraine effects may be the result of calcium channel blockade.[40]

Bille et al. treated 19 children with cyproheptadine for 3 to 6 months in an uncontrolled trial.[39] Seventeen of the 19 children had improvement in their headache frequency, and 4 of 17 had resolution of their headaches. Dosages used ranged from 0.2 to 0.4 mg per kg per day. Although this was an uncontrolled study in a small number of children, this dosage of cyproheptadine has been quoted in several medical texts and review articles as appropriate for migraine prevention.

Cyproheptadine can be used as a single daily dosage administered at bedtime, starting at 2 to 4 mg per day (see Table 6–11). The vast majority of patients respond to a dosage between 4 and 12 mg per day. The antihistaminic effects of cyproheptadine may cause significant sedation. Weight gain, drowsiness, and dry mouth, as well as irritability, also can occur.[23]

β-Blockers

The β-blockers may exert their effect through antagonism of the $5\text{-}HT_2$ receptors or through modulation of adrenoreceptors. The evidence that propranolol is effective in migraine prophylaxis is very weak, yet propranolol remains a mainstay in the preventive treatment of migraine headaches in children.

Dosing of propranolol (Inderal) has not been systemically studied. Ludvigsson studied 28 children with dosages ranging from 60 mg per day, for children weighing less than 35 kg, to 120 mg per day, for children weighing greater than 35 kg.[41] He concluded that a dose of 1 mg per kg per day is effective. Olness et al., in a study comparing self-hypnosis to propranolol for the treatment of classic migraine headache, used a dosage of 3 mg per kg per day.[42] They found that self-hypnosis was more efficacious than propranolol in reducing headache frequency. Neither self-hypnosis nor propranolol affected subjective or objective measures of headache severity. Forsythe et al. suggested that propranolol had no impact on frequency of migraine headache and may have increased the duration of headache in some children.[43] The final dosage per kilogram used in that study is not reported. The recommended starting dosage of propranolol for the treatment of hypertension in children is 1 mg per kg per day up to 10 mg twice daily. The dosage can be titrated slowly, increasing over 2 to 4 weeks to a maximum of 3 to 4 mg per kg per day divided twice daily, if tolerated (see Table 6–11).[23] Adolescents may experience significant drops in blood pressure and, consequently, develop the "weak and dizzies." The β-blockers can also reduce stamina and should be used with caution in athletes. Propranolol is contraindicated in children with a prior history of reactive airway disease or diabetes and in some children with cardiac arrhythmia. Although the majority of children have no significant side effects from propranolol, several side effects can occur including fatigue, nausea, dizziness, vivid dreams, insomnia, nightmares, depression, and memory disturbance. One of the most significant side effects, which easily can be missed in an adolescent, is the onset of depression. Patients should be monitored for signs of mild depression within the first 4 to 8 weeks of therapy initiation; the signs may be subtle. If depression symptoms are observed, the dose may need to be decreased or discontinued. If a child experiences nightmares or vivid dreams while taking propranolol, changing the dosing schedule so that the child receives the medication several hours before retiring usually eliminates that side effect.[23] In spite of the potential for side effects, most children tolerate propranolol well.

Patients should be evaluated at approximately 4 and 12 weeks into the treatment phase to determine if the medication has been effective and well tolerated. It is important to remember that the β-blockers may take several weeks to have their full effect. A minimum of 12 weeks of treatment at appropriate doses is needed to determine if the medication has been efficacious.

Although other β-blockers have been used clinically for several years, there are no studies to demonstrate their usefulness in children. Norohna reported that the β-blocker timolol is not effective as a preventive medication in children.[44] However, this was a very small study involving only 17 children. Nadolol has been reported to be as equally efficacious as propranolol in adult studies.[45] However, the data must be interpreted with respect to the assessment of Ramadan et al. concerning the scientific merit of many of these studies.[46] Propranolol (Inderal) and timolol maleate (Blocadren) have been approved by the FDA for the treatment of migraine prevention (see Table 6–12).

Calcium Channel Blockers

Calcium channel blockers have been used quite extensively in the adult population.[47] Flunarizine, a calcium channel blocker available in Europe but not in the United States, has been shown to be effective as a preventive medication in children.[48–52] In the double-blind, placebo-controlled crossover study performed by Sorge et al., patients were crossed over from active drug to placebo following a 4-month active treatment phase.[48] The baseline mean number of headache attacks per month was 3 for both groups. In the flunarizine-treated group, the mean number of attacks per month decreased progressively to a low of 1.3 per month. Thus, the actual change in headache number was small but statistically significant. No data are presented beyond 4 months; thus, it is unknown if treatment beyond that point would have demonstrated a continued clinical efficacy. All studies of flunarizine report similar outcomes.[49–52]

The efficacy of flunarizine should not be generalized to suggest that all calcium channel blockers will be effective. Only nimodipine, a class-2 (nifedipine-like) calcium entry blocker for slow calcium channels, has been reported to reduce the frequency of migraine headache in children.[53] However, in the first phase of this double-blind, placebo-controlled crossover trial there was an identical reduction in headache frequency in both the placebo and the active drug group. After crossover, the initial placebo group responded to nimodipine with a reduction in headache frequency greater than the second placebo group. The authors conclude that nimodipine is efficacious as a migraine preventive agent. However, the data do not appear to support their conclusions.

Clinical experience suggests that calcium channel blockers are not any more efficacious than other classes of agents. Calcium channel blocker side effects include constipation, hypotension, AV block, nausea, weight gain, and occasionally, depression. The side effects of the calcium channel blockers may prove limiting in some patients.

Nonsteroidal Anti-inflammatory Drugs

The NSAIDs, such as naproxen sodium, are known to be efficacious in the treatment of acute migraine headache and have been reported to be effective as a migraine preventive medication.

Lewis et al. treated 19 children with naproxen sodium, 250 mg twice daily, in a double-blind, placebo-controlled crossover trial.[54] Ten of the 19 patients completed the study, and of these 10, 6 reported a significant reduction in frequency and severity of their headaches. Of the 6, 3 reported a 50% reduction in headache frequency, 2 a greater than 70% reduction, and 1 a greater than 90% reduction. Thus, this relatively small study suggests that naproxen sodium may be effective.

Our clinical experience indicates that naproxen sodium is an effective preventive medication. A starting dosage of 10 mg per kg twice daily reduces migraine headache frequency and lessens the severity of breakthrough headaches. Long-term use of NSAIDs may not be advisable because of their effects on the gut and on renal function. However, for some patients who have difficulty tolerating the other treatments, this may be a reasonable short-term alternative for up to 4 to 8 weeks.

Other Agents

Single reports on the use of trazodone and pizotifen in a small number of children suggest that these agents may be effective in preventing migraine.[55,56] However, no confirmatory data are available. Clonidine has been studied in a single double-blind, placebo-controlled trial involving 57 children. There was no significant difference in headache frequency between treatment and placebo groups. Clonidine was most helpful in a subset of patients with visual aura or a positive family history of migraine.

Ergotamine compounds, such as methylergonovine maleate (Methergine) and methysergide, have not been studied in the adolescent or pediatric population. Because of their long-term potential to cause retroperitoneal fibrosis, their use, even in the adult population, is somewhat limited.

Treatment Period

A difficult and unanswered question is how long should a patient be treated with preventive medication? A survey by the Pediatric Committee of the American Headache Society, formally the American Association for the Study of Headache, was unable to reach a consensus in this regard (personal communications between Dr. Wasiewski and the Pediatric Committee of the American Headache Society, 1998).[19] Treatment periods with preventive medication typically range from as short as 3 months to as long

Table 6–13   Parents' Approach to Children's Headache

< 11 years — reinforce symptom-free intervals while using distracting supportive comments or by selectively ignoring pain-related behavior

> 11 years — provide supportive and empathic responses to headache-related behavior

Adapted from: Lewis DW, et al. Pediatric headache: what do the children want? Headache 1996;36:224–230.

Table 6–14   Successful Management of Pediatric Headache

Reassure patient and parents there is no central nervous system lesion.

Educate patients and their parents about the pathogenesis and natural history of migraine.

Establish realistic goals for treatment according to age.

as 18 months, with 6 months being the mean. Committee members have agreed that withdrawing medication during the school year is not advisable. Treatment periods of 6 to 12 months generally result in a significant reduction in frequency and a persistent effect after withdrawal of preventive medication. Children started on preventive medications in the beginning of the school year should continue the medications throughout the school year, in general. If significant headache control has been achieved, the medication may be withdrawn preferably the following summer. If, on the other hand, the children's medication is begun late in the school year, it may be discontinued either through a prolonged break or through the following year and withdrawn the following summer depending on the clinical situation.

The management of migraine in children and adolescents should include a discussion of the therapeutic goals with both the patients and their parents (Tables 6–13 and 6–14).[25,57]

CONCLUSION

Medication options are improving for both children and adolescents with regard to the acute treatment and the preventive management of migraine. The combined use of pharmacologic and nonpharmacologic modalities can prove to be quite efficacious in the complete relief of migraine headaches in this patient population.

REFERENCES

1. Sillanpaa M. Changes in the prevalence of migraine and other headaches during the first seven school years. Headache 1983;23:15–19.
2. Gladstein J, Holden EW, Peralta L, Raven M. Diagnoses and symptom patterns in children presenting to a pediatric headache clinic. Headache 1993,33:497–500.
3. Seshia SS, Wolstein JR, Adams C, et al. International Headache Society criteria and childhood headache. Dev Med Child Neurol 1994;36:419–428.
4. Winner P, Martinez W, Mate L, Bello L. Classification of pediatric migraine: proposed revision of the IHS criteria. Headache 1995;35:407–410.
5. Winner P, Gladstein S, Hamel R, et al. Multicenter prospective evauation of proposed pediatric migraine revisions to the IHS criteria. Presented at the American Association for the Study of Headache scientific meeting, San Diego, CA, May 1996.
6. Hamalainen M, Hoppu K, Santavuori P. Sumatriptan for migraine attacks in children: a randomized, placebo-controlled study. Do children with migraine respond to oral sumpatriptan differently from adults? Neurology 1997;48:1100–1103.
7. Aromaa M, Rautava P, Helenius H, Sillanpaa ML. Factors of early life as predictors of headache in children at school entry. Headache 1998;38:23–30.
8. Linder SL. Subcutaneous sumatriptan in the clinical setting. The first 50 consecutive patients with acute migraine in a pediatric neurology office practice. Headache 1996;36:419–422.
9. Winner P, Pensky A, Linder S. Efficacy and safety of oral sumatriptan in adolescent migraines. Presented at the American Association for the Study of Headache scientific meeting, Chicago, IL, May 1996.
10. Winner P, Rothner AD, Saper J, et al. Sumatriptan nasal spray in the treatment of acute migraine in adolescent. Pediatrics (in press).
11. MacDonald J. Treatment of juvenile migraine with subcutaneous sumatriptan. Headache 1994;34:581–582.
12. Diamond S, Elkind A, Jackson R, et al. Multiple-attack efficacy and tolerability of sumatriptan nasal spray in the treatment of migraine. Arch Fam Med 1998;7:234–240.
13. Ryan R, Elkind A, Baker C, et al. Sumatriptan nasal spray for the acute treatment of migraine. Results of two clinical studies. Neurology 1997;49:1225–1230.
14. Schoenen J, Bulcke J, Caebeke J. Self-treatment of acute migraine with subcutaneous sumatriptan using an auto-injector device: comparison with customary treatment in an open, longitudinal study. Cephalalgia 1994;14:55–63.

15. Winner P. Clinical profile of rizatriptan 5 mg in adolescent migraineurs. Presented at the American Academy of Neurology annual meeting, San Diego, CA, April 2000.

16. Linder SL, Dowson AJ. Zolmitriptan provides effective migraine relief in adolescents. Int J Clin Prac 2000;54:466–469.

17. Horton BT, Peters GA, Blumenthal LS. A new product in the treatment of migraine; a preliminary report. Mayo Clin Proc 1945;20:241–248.

18. Raskin NH. Repetitive intravenous dihydroergotamine as therapy for intra migraine. Neurology 1986;36:995–997.

19. Winner P, Ricalde O, Le Force B, et al. A double-blind study of subcutaneous dihydroergotamine vs subcutaneous sumatriptan in the treatment of acute migraine. Arch Neurol 1996;53:180–184.

20. Linder SL. Treatment of childhood headache with dihydroergotamine mesylate. Headache 1994;34:578–580.

21. Linder SL. Treatment of acute childhood migraine headaches. Cephalalgia 1991;11(Suppl II):120–121.

22. Practice parameter: appropriate use of ergotamine tartrate and dihydroergotamine in the treatment of migraine and status migrainosus (summary statement). Report of the Quality Standards Subcommittee of the American Academy of Neurology. Neurology 1995;45:585–587.

23. Winner P, Visser WH, Lines CR. Headaches in children. Postgrad Med 1995; 101(5):81–90.

24. Riback PS. Factors precipitating migraine headache in children. Ann Neurol 1999;46:541.

25. Winner P. Pediatric headaches: what's new? Curr Opin Neurol 1999;12:269–272.

26. Goadsby PS. How do currently used prophylactic agents work in migraine? Cephalalgia 1997;17:85–92.

27. Klapper J. Divalproex sodium in migraine prophylaxis: a dose-controlled study. Cephalalgia 1997:17:103–108.

28. Cutrer FM, Limmroth V, Moskowitz VA. Possible mechanisms of valproate in migraine prophylaxis. Cephalalgia 1997;17:93–100.

29. Hernig-Hanit R. Baclofen for prevention of migraine. Cephalalgia 1999;19:589–591.

30. Diamond S, Ryan RE, Klappel JA, et al. Dotarizine in the prophylaxis of migraine headaches. Headache 1999;39:350.

31. Edwards KR, Santarcangelo V. Intravenous valpropate for acute treatment of migraine headache. Headache 1999;39:353.

32. Freitag F, Saper J, Winner P, Collins D. Depakote ER in migraine prophylaxis. Presented at the 52nd annual meeting of the American Academy of Neurology, Montreal, Canada, May 1, 2000.

33. Caruso JM, Ferri R, Exil G, et al. The efficacy of divalproex sodium in the pro-phylactic treatment of migraine. Ann Neurol 1998;44:567.

34. Matthew N, Saper J, Silberstein S, et al. Migraine prophylaxis with divalproex. Arch Neurol 1995;52:281–286.

35. Silberstein S. Divalproex sodium in headache: literature review and clinical guidelines. Headache 1996;9:547–555.

36. Hershey AD, Powers SW, Brenntti AL, et al. Standard dosing of amitriptyline is highly effective in a pediatric headache center population. Headache 1999;39:357–358.

37. Levinstein B. A comparative study of cyproheptadine, amitriptyline, and pro-pranolol in the treatment of adolescent migraine. Cephalalgia 1991;11 (Suppl 11):122–123.

38. Adly C, Straumanis J, Chesson A. Fluoxetine prophylaxis of migraine. Headache 1992;32:101–104.

39. Bille B, Ludvigsson J, Sanner G. Prophylaxis of migraine in children. Headache 1977:17:61–63.

40. Peroutka SJ, Allen GS. The calcium antagonist properties of cypropheptadine: implications for anti-migraine action. Neurology 1984;34:304–309.

41. Ludvigsson J. Propranolol used in prophylaxis of migraine in children. Acta Neurol Scand 1974;50:109–115.

42. Olness K, MacDonald JT, Ulden DL. Comparison of self-hypnosis and propra-nolol in treatment of juvenile class migraine. Pediatrics 1987;79:593–597.

43. Forsythe JI, Gillies D, Sills MA. Propanolol ('Inderal') in treatment of child-hood migraine. Dev Med Child Neurol 1984:26:737–741.

44. Noronha MJ. Double-blind randomized cross-over trial of timolol in migraine prophylaxis in children. Cephalalgia 1985;5(Suppl 3):174–175.

45. Olerud B, Gustausson CL, Furberg B. Nadolol and propranolol in migraine management. Headache 1986;26:490–493.

46. Ramadan NM, Shultz LL, Gilkey SJ. Migraine prophylactic drugs: proof of efficacy, utilization and cost. Cephalalgia 1997;17:73–78.

47. Toda N, Tfelt-Hansen P. Calcium antagonists. In Oleson J, Tfelt-Hansen P, Welch KMA, eds. The Headaches. New York, NY: Raven Press, 1993, pp 383–390.

48. Sorge F, DeSimone R, Marano E, et al. Flunarizine in prophylaxis of child-hood migraine. Cephalalgia 1988:8:1–6.

49. Pothman R. Calcium-antagonist flunarizine vs. low-dose acetylsalicyclic acid in children migraine—a double-blind study. Cephalalgia 1987;7(Suppl 6): 385–386.

50. Martinez-Lage JM. Flunarizine (Sibelium) in the prophylaxis of migraine. An open, long-term multicenter trial. Cephalalgia 1988;8(Suppl 8):15–20.

51. Sorge F, Marano E. Flunarizine v. placebo in childhood migraine. A double-blind study. Cephalalgia 1985;5(Suppl 2):145–148.

52. Guidetti V, Moscato D, Ottauiano S, et al. Flunarizine and migraine in childhood. Cephalalgia 1987;7:263–266.

53. Battistella PA, Ruffilli R, Moro R, et al. A placebo-controlled crossover trial of nimodipine in pediatric migraine. Headache 1990;30:264–268.

54. Lewis DW, Middlebrook M, Mehallick M, et al. Naproxen for migraine prophylaxis. Ann Neurol 1994;36:542.

55. Salmon M. Pizotifen (B.C. 105 Sandomigran) in prophylaxis of childhood migraine. Headache 1995;35:174.

56. Battistella PA, Ruffilli R, Cernetti R, et al. A placebo-controlled crossover trial using trazodone in pediatric migraine. Headache 1993;33:36–39.

57. Lewis DW, Middlebrook MT, Mehallick L, et al. Pediatric headache: what do the children want? Headache 1996;36:224–230.

Chapter 7

Chronic Daily Headache

Jack Gladstein and Paul Winner

O f those adults with chronic daily headache (CDH), 23% report that the onset of their headache was intermittent before age 9, and 36% from ages 10 to 19.[1] Adults have reported a gradual transition from intermittent headaches into daily headaches over an average of 10.7 years. Studies in children and adolescents are important to help us understand and advance the knowledge of CDH in all age groups.

Chronic daily headache is a diagnostic term describing a patient who suffers from recurrent headaches averaging 15 days per month and who does not have an underlying serious medical condition. It was described in adults by Mathew et al. in 1987.[2] Estimating incidence and prevalence of this disorder has been difficult since strict uniform definitions have not been formed. Nevertheless, the prevalence rate for severe or recurrent headache in children and adolescents has been reported as 0.2%, 0.8%, and 2.5% by Newachek et al.,[3] Sillanpaa et al.,[4] and Abu-Arafeh and Russell,[5] respectively. For the sufferers and their families, this condition is a source of concern and disability. It may mask depression and cause a tremendous amount of dysfunction for youngsters and their families. In this chapter we will present the data known about this condition and offer an approach to rational diagnosis and treatment.

CLASSIFICATION

In adults, Mathew et al.[2] described CDH as chronic recurrent headache that transformed from either episodic migraine or tension-type headache. Solomon et al.[6] in 1992 and Messinger et al.[7] in 1991 attempted to use the International Headache Society criteria to classify consecutive adults in their series but were not able to in over one-third of cases. This led to the work of Silberstein et al.[8] in 1994 who defined four types of CDH, each with or without medication overuse (Table 7–1). In their proposed criteria, a person has transformed migraine (chronic migraine) if she/he had a history of episodic migraine that has now become a daily or near daily experience. Headache duration is greater than 4 hours per day, and this progression with increasing frequency and decreasing severity occurs over at least 3 months.

With chronic tension-type headache, the patient has an average headache frequency of 15 days per month (180 days per year) for 6 months. The headache has two of the following pain characteristics: a pressing/tightening quality, bilateral location, mild or moderate severity, not aggravated by walking stairs or similar routine physical activity, and no autonomic characteristics. There is also a history of episodic tension-type headache. Again there is a transformation period of at least 3 months.

With new persistent daily headache, the symptoms may begin in childhood or adolescence as an acute onset of constant unremitting headache that develops over less than 3 days. A history of evaluation is absent. The headache lasts more than 4 hours per day and is more frequent than 15 times per month.

With hemicrania continua, headaches are unilateral and continuous with reported fluctuations in pain intensity. There is a female preponderance, which may start in adolescence. Autonomic features (i.e., conjunctival injection, lacrimation, nasal congestion, rhinorrhea, ptosis, eyelid edema) are associated with exacerbations of pain. Hemicrania continua headaches present for at least 1 month and are treated with indomethacin.

We attempted to apply these criteria to a consecutive cohort of children and adolescents who presented to a tertiary referral clinic in 1996.[9] We found that 45% of children and adolescents in our population did not

Table 7–1   Silberstein's Classification of Chronic Daily Headache

Transformed migraine

Chronic tension-type headache

New persistent daily headache

Hemicrania continua

Adapted from: Silberstein SD, Lipton RB, Solomon S, Mathew NT. Classification of daily and near-daily headaches: proposed revisions to the HIS criteria. Headache 1994;34:1–7.

fit neatly into these categories. By adding a category we called the "comorbid" (migraine and tension-type headache, mixed headache), all but one of our 37 patients could be classified according to Silberstein et al.'s 1994 criteria. In this type, it is as if two headache patterns exist independently of each other, without any transformation. There is an underlying tension-type headache, with intermittent full blown migraine. In 1996, Silberstein et al. made modifications by loosening the diagnostic criteria for transformed migraine (chronic migraine) and thereby, capturing a lot of their patients with comorbid headache (mixed headache).[10] We have continued with the 1994 criteria because we feel that the lack of transformation in so many of our youngsters merits a separate category for those with comorbid headache (mixed headache).

Currently, the Pediatric Committee of the American Headache Society is attempting to classify CDH with a questionnaire used in 15 sites across the country. Findings are preliminary at this point.

Case Presentation: A 16-year-old girl in the eleventh grade has a long history of headaches. Her headaches started at age 9 but only occurred four times a year. They were bilateral and came to peak intensity in 1 hour. Although she had no aura, she had a feeling that they were coming back because of excessive tiredness about 1 hour before headache onset. Her headache back then was throbbing. It had accompanied photophobia and phonophobia. She lost her appetite but denied nausea or vomiting. These headaches lasted for about 2 hours and responded to acetaminophen. While her headache was in full force she needed to lie down in a dark room and was unable to read or exercise.

Over the years, her individual headaches were similar, but their frequency increased gradually. For the past year, she has developed a pattern of daily or near daily headaches where, routinely, she complains of bilateral pain with little in the way of autonomic symptoms, as before, that made her go and lie down until the next morning.

Her past medical history is noncontributory. Her mother and father suffer with "sinus headaches." Her older sister is away at college, whereas she lives at home with her parents. She is an "A" student and active in the drama club. She denies the use of medications, drugs, alcohol, or cigarettes. She denies sexual activity.

This patient's history is most consistent with CDH: transformed migraine (chronic migraine). What are some of the aspects of this patient's history that may help us design a treatment plan? Does she get more headaches around the time of her drama club performances? Yes.

This patient does meet criteria for preventive treatment due to functional disability. She was treated with an oral triptan for her acute migraine attacks and was placed on daily preventive medication. She also received relaxation training, which reportedly was helpful in controlling her daily headaches

Now we will discuss the controversial nature of this topic and point out some of differences between children/adolescents and adults.

HISTORY

For patients with chronic headache, as with all patients, a skilled and careful history is the most important step in making the diagnosis and preparing a plan of action. To get to the diagnosis of CDH, serious medical diseases must be ruled out and then an attempt must be made to give the diagnosis a name. We use the 1994 Silberstein et al. criteria[8] with the addition of comorbid pattern (mixed headache) for those youngsters who have underlying tension-type headache with independent superimposed migraine. While obtaining a careful headache history to rule out chronic illness or tumor, coping mechanisms and disability should be explored.[11] For adolescent headache sufferers, it is critical to interview the youngster and parent(s) together and separately. By having them start the interview together, the practitioner gains critical information about how they interact. Does the mother answer all the questions for the teen? Is there a lot of conflict? By separating them later, we learn about what each person perceives to be the problem and the disability, and we show to all involved the practitioner's endorsement of their views. If the youngster will not separate or if the parent will not let go, we learn a lot about the problem. By bringing the parties together at the end of the session, we can then summarize the situation, while not betraying anyone's confidence. This approach takes time, so patients with chronic headache often require increased scheduling time by office staff, if possible.

While obtaining the history, the practitioner must discuss symptoms and disability and rule out the possibility of infections, sinus disease, trauma, hypertension, cerebrospinal pressure abnormalities, ocular disorders, and factitious disorders or somatization.[12] A careful look at psychosocial factors is crucial as well. Dietary, sleep, and medication histories may help pinpoint aggravating factors. A family history of headache and/or psychiatric disease may shed additional light on the problem. Psychiatric comorbidity of depression or anxiety disorders has been reported to occur more frequently in the patient with CDH than in the patient with migraine or intermittent tension-type headache alone.[13] The presence or absence of daily medication overuse plays a big part in treatment options. Assessing disability for a youngster can be measured primarily by days of school missed, days of school requiring early dismissal, visits to nurses for medication, a drop in grades, and/or an inability to participate in after-school activities. Disparity between parent- and patient-endorsed severity is suspicious for either child-parent conflict or parental overestimation of symptoms. In the younger child, one gleans helpful information from a careful description of how the parents react to the child when headache is acknowledged. "Is all okay at home?" and "What is your home like?" are open-ended questions to be answered by the youngster and the parents separately.

PHYSICAL EXAMINATION

The approach to the youngster with chronic headache demands a thorough physical examination to convince both the practitioner and the patient of a benign etiology before proceeding with a treatment plan. Having the patient undressed will facilitate a good dermatologic examination and the ability to assess Tanner staging in the adolescent. Vital signs help rule out increased intracranial pressure as well as hypertension. A skin examination helps rule out neurofibromatosis as well as tuberous sclerosis. Palpation of the sinuses and the jaw help to rule out sinusitis and temporomandibular joint (TMJ) disorders, respectively. A careful neurologic examination should include a check of visual fields and a funduscopic examination. Emphasizing normalcy along the way makes the examination a teaching experience for the youngster. A thorough mental status examination may help diagnose depression or somatization. When there is mood incongruence, a patient may describe horrific symptoms but show "la belle indifférence."

PHYSIOLOGY

There is much literature regarding the physiology of migraine; however studies related to the etiology and physiology of tension-type headache have been more sparse. There are no studies that look at the physiology of CDH as an entity by itself; they focus on recurrent migraine or tension-type headache. Nevertheless, in tension-type headache, patients have been shown to respond to stress with stronger muscle contraction than nonheadache sufferers.[14] Jensen et al. suggested that prolonged muscle contraction may sensitize the central nervous system to a lower general sensitivity to pain.[15]

ETIOLOGIC FACTORS

The role of stress has been considered an important factor in chronic headache since the work of Bille in 1962.[16] Stress has been shown to be more common in headache sufferers than in matched controls.[17] Bille[16] pointed out, and many headache centers report, that school stress–induced headaches are gone in the summertime. Anxiety, depression, and chronic somatic complaints are more common in headache sufferers; however we don't know if the headaches cause the other complaints or if the complaints are a consequence of having longstanding headaches.[18] It is interesting to note, however, that various psychologic symptoms are only elevated when a subject has a headache at the time of measurement, so data interpretation of such studies may be biased by the intensity of pain.[9,19]

Familial patterns of headache do exist, especially for recurrent migraine.[20] Familial aggregation is lower in tension-type headache.[21] More important than family history is the response of the family to headache behavior, which may influence the transformation from an acute to a chronic condition.[22]

DIAGNOSTIC WORKUP

Patients with suspicious histories or abnormal physical findings need an appropriate workup. For patients with growth delay or pubertal delay or arrest, a medical workup is indicated. For patients with dermatologic examinations that are suspicious for a neurocutaneous disorder, brain imaging is indicated (magnetic resonance imaging with and without contrast preferred). Sinus tenderness (computed tomography scan of the sinuses) or painful, limited jaw opening may warrant further dental investigation. Most patients with CDH have been imaged at some point as their headache progression went from acute to chronic. The exception would be those patients with new persistent daily headache, where the chronic headache started at the onset. Studies of children with recurrent headache who have no significant change in the severity or frequency of the headache over the prior 4 months and an absence of physical examination abnormalities do not require further imaging.[23] Electroencephalograms are similarly not helpful in the vast majority of cases unless there is a history of an atypical aura or concern of a paroxysmal event.[24]

TREATMENT

The treatment of CDH in children and adolescents remains empiric since few good studies have been done. A rational approach based on careful consideration of headache type, the presence or absence of medication overuse, and functional disability will assure that patients get judicious treatment. Assessment of a youngster's ability to comply with relaxation training will help optimize outcome, since only those youngsters who practice the relaxation training will succeed.

For patients with daily headache, it is important to find out whether they have intermittent migraine-like headaches on top of the chronic tension-type headache (mixed headache). Those with migraines can be treated with appropriate acute management. Careful instruction in these medications will aim to prevent inappropriate use of these powerful agents (see acute treatment strategies in Chapter 6). The presence of daily medication (overuse) makes treatment more complicated. Abrupt withdrawal of these medications will precipitate severe headache. Therefore, the practitioner must be cautious in recommending cessation until some preventive measure is in place.

Although there are many studies demonstrating efficacy of preventive agents in adults, few well-designed, controlled studies have been performed specifically in children. Even fewer have been done with CDH. Nevertheless, there are childhood studies or combinations of adult and adolescent studies using β-blockers,[25–27] tricyclic antidepressants,[28] calcium channel blockers,[29] and valproate.[30] Studies on this subject do not rigorously define chronic headache, so treatment at this point is quite

Table 7–2	Management of Chronic Daily Headache
Pharmacologic	Stress management
Acute treatment	Elimination of triggers
Preventive treatment	Regular sleep patterns
Biofeedback	Regular exercise

empiric. Nevertheless, practitioners have been using these medications for years (see preventive therapy strategies in Chapter 6).

Behavioral treatment shows promise for patients with chronic headache.[31] Obvious advantages include the absence of medication side effects and helping youngsters gain mastery of their chronic pain. The disadvantages are in patient selection. Behavioral treatment does not work if it is not practiced regularly. Therefore, the practitioner must know the patient's lifestyle and ability to comply with the daily practice routine. We have found that the best candidates are those who are the most busy already. They find the time to practice, whereas the patient whose life is in chaos will not comply. For both behavioral and pharmacologic prevention of recurrent headache, no study has used rigorous definitions of headache type. We do not know, for instance, if patients with chronic tension-type headache respond differently from patients with transformed migraine (chronic migraine) or comorbid headache (mixed headache) (Table 7–2).

PROGNOSIS

Although Bille's classic study had a 40-year follow-up, there is no study specifically looking at patients with CDH who started in their childhood or adolescent years.

CONCLUSION

The study of CDH in children and adolescents is in its nascent stages. With a rigorous classification scheme, we now have the possibility of multicenter studies to elucidate whether the clinical patterns seen by experienced observers translate into rational differentiation of treatment approaches. If the entities are indeed different, then therapeutic, prophylactic, and behavioral trials could guide us in offering a more evidence-based approach to the treatment of this fascinating yet sometimes debilitating condition.

REFERENCES

1. Spierings ELH, Schroevara M, Honkoop PC, Sorbi M. Development of chronic daily headache: a clinical study. Headache 1998;38:529–533.
2. Mathew NT, Reuveni U, Perez F. Transformed or evolutive migraine. Headache 1987;27:102–106.
3. Newachek PW, Taylor WR. Childhood chronic illness: prevalence, severity, and impact. Am J Public Health 1992;82:364–371.
4. Sillanpaa M, Piekkala P, Kero P. Prevalence of headache in preschool age in an unselected child population. Cephalalgia 1991;11:239–242.
5. Abu-Arafeh I, Russell G. Prevalence of headache and migraine in school children. BMJ 1994;34:508–514.
6. Solomon S, Lipton RB, Newman LC. Evaluation of chronic daily headache—comparison to criteria for chronic tension-type headache. Cephalalgia 1992;12:365–368.
7. Messinger HB, Spierings ELH, Vincent AJP. Overlap of migraine and tension-type headache in the International Headache Society classification. Cephalalgia 1991;11:233–237.
8. Silberstein SD, Lipton RB, Solomon S, Mathew NT. Classification of daily and near-daily headaches: proposed revisions to the HIS criteria. Headache 1994;34:1–7.
9. Gladstein J. Holden EW. Chronic daily headache in children and adolescents: a 2-year prospective study. Headache 1996;36:349–351.
10. Silberstein SD, Lipton RB, Sliwinski M. Classification of daily and near-daily headaches: field trial of revised IHS criteria. Neurology 1996;47:871–875.
11. Holden EW, Levy JD, Deichmann MM, Gladstein J. Recurrent pediatric headaches: assessment and intervention. J Dev Behav Pediatr 1998;19:109–116.
12. Gladstein J, Holden EW, Winner P, et al. Chronic daily headache in children and adolescents: current status and recommendations for the future. Headache 1997;37:626–629.
13. Guidetti V, Galli F, Fabrizi P, et al. Headache and psychiatric comorbidity: clinical aspects and outcome in an 8-year follow-up study. Cephalalgia 1998;18:455–462.
14. Martin PR. Psychological Management of Chronic Headaches. New York: Guilford Press, 1993.

15. Jensen R, Berndtsen L, Olesen J. Muscular factors are of importance in tension-type headache. Headache 1998;38:10–17.

16. Bille B. Migraine in school children. Acta Paediatr Scand 1962;51(Suppl 136):1–151.

17. Larsson BS. The role of psychological, health behaviour and medical factors in adolescent headache. Dev Med Child Neurol 1988;30:616–625.

18. Larsson B. Recurrent headaches in children and adeolescents. In: McGrath PJ, Finley GA, eds. Chronic and Recurrent Pain in Children and Adolescents. Progress in Pain Research and Management: 13. Seattle: IASP Press, 1999, pp 115–140.

19. Holroyd KA, France JL, Nash JM, Hursey KG. Pain state as artifact in the psychological assessment of recurrent headache sufferers. Pain 1993;53: 229–235.

20. Ziegler DK, Hur Y-Mi, Bouchard TJ, et al. Migraine in twins raised together and apart. Headache 1998;38:417–422.

21. Metsahonkala L, Sillanpaa M, Touminen J. Outcome of early school age migraine. Cephalalgia 1997;17:662–665.

22. Wall BA, Holden EW, Gladstein J. Parent responses to pediatric headache. Headache 1997;37:65–70.

23. Chu ML, Shinnar S. Headaches in children younger than 7 years of age. Arch Neurol 1992;49:79–82.

24. Daly DD, Markland OM. Focal brain lesion. In: Daly DD, Pedley TA, eds. Current Practice of Clinical Electroencephelography. New York: Raven Press, 1990.

25. Ludvigsson J. Propranolol used in prophylaxis of migraine in children. Acta Neurol Scand 1974;50:109–115.

26. Forsythe WI, Gillies D, Sills MA. Propranolol ('Inderal') in the treatment of childhood migraine. Dev Med Child Neurol 1984;26:737–741.

27. Olness K. MacDonald JT, Uden DL. Comparison of self-hypnosis and propranolol in the treatment of juvenile classic migraine. Pediatrics 1984;79:593–597.

28. Diamond S, Baltes BJ. Chronic tension headache—treated with amitriptyline—a double blind study. Headache 1971;11:110–116.

29. Solomon GD. The action and uses of calcium channel blockers in migraine and cluster headache. Headache 1990;10:111–116.

30. Sorensen KV. Valproate: a new drug in migraine prophylaxis. Acta Neurol Scand 1988;78:346–348.

31. Engel JM, Rapoff MA, Pressman AR. Long-term follow-up of relaxation training for pediatric headache disorders. Headache 1992;32:152–156.

Chapter 8

PSYCHOLOGIC AND NONPHARMACOLOGIC TREATMENT OF HEADACHE

Donald W. Lewis
and Alvin E. Lake III

When a family presents to the primary care provider for the medical evaluation of their child's headache, there are always interwoven psychologic aspects. The parents dreadfully fear that their child has a brain tumor. The young patient may be experiencing limitations in his or her lifestyle and curtailing activities or school attendance, which in turn leads to secondary affective disturbances. The headache itself may be a manifestation of internal or external emotional stressors from school, parents, or classmates. As discussed in Chapter 3, a thorough history is essential not only to determine the cause of the headache but also to delineate the presence of predisposing or aggravating factors that must be addressed for a successful treatment to be realized.

The purpose of this chapter is to review the nonpharmacologic and psychologic treatment strategies and options available for children and adolescents with headache.

CONFIDENT REASSURANCE

First and foremost in the family's mind is a fear that their child's headache may be indicative of serious neurologic disease. Very likely, the child harbors these same concerns. In a survey of children presenting to a pediatric headache clinic, the following question was asked: "What do you want from your visit to the doctor?" Their responses revealed three key concerns: What was the cause of the headache?, What will make it better?, and Are they going to die?[1]

Children as young as 5 or 6 years old reported an overwhelming fear that their headaches could be due to brain tumors, a thought planted by parents, siblings, television, or movies. As part of the survey, the children were asked to draw their headache. Their drawings, analyzed by an art therapist, disclosed striking depressive features, particularly among teenaged boys, in whom over 50% depicted themselves as dead or dying.

After careful medical history and physical examination and before any treatment regimen can be rationally considered, the physician must answer the children's three questions in a straightforward manner. The physician must explain to them what is causing their headache, outline the plan of treatment, and confidently reassure both the children and their families that there are no signs of tumors or other serious neurologic diseases.

A common error made by well-meaning caregivers is to summarize by saying, "I don't think there is anything bad going on." This kind of innocent remark generally heightens the patient's anxiety.

NONPHARMACOLOGIC MANAGEMENT

The family and patient must understand that pharmacologic and nonpharmacologic measures are equally important in the treatment of headache. Several well-designed trials of behavioral or psychologic treatments have demonstrated their effectiveness.[2] A meta-analysis of behavioral versus pharmacologic interventions for pediatric migraine found psychologic interventions to be successful in decreasing the frequency of migraine attacks.[3] In fact, given the paucity of validated research in pediatric headache, behavioral treatments have been more convincingly documented to have efficacy than many of the commonly used drug regimens described in Chapter 6.[4] In a head-to-head comparison study using relaxation training with stress management versus the β-blocker metoprolol, behavioral therapy was significantly more effective in reducing headache frequency, intensity, and duration than β-blockers for pediatric migraine.[5] The value of these techniques must not be underestimated.

The majority of research into psychologic interventions for childhood headache have included mixed populations with tension-type headache and migraine. Those studies that have targeted a specific headache subset have focused on childhood migraine. Therefore, generalization of the results to all pediatric headache must be done with caution.[6] A subset of children and adolescents who may potentially benefit from these modalities more than any other is the chronic daily headache group. Unfortunately, published research into treatments of this group of patients, either pharmacologic or psychologic, is minimal.

A variety of strategies are available to prevent or decrease the frequency of headaches when patients are experiencing numerous attacks or when their headaches have evolved to a daily or near daily pattern. We have chosen to divide these strategies into (1) avoiding analgesic overuse, (2) lifestyle modifications, (3) behavioral therapies, (4) the addressing of school issues, and (5) individual and family therapy.

Avoiding Analgesic Overuse

The excessive use of either nonprescription or prescription analgesics and abortives has a demonstrated role in the transformation of intermittent migraine to chronic daily headache and interferes with the effectiveness of both prophylactic pharmacotherapy and nonpharmacologic treatment.[7] The advice to take pain medication as soon as the pain begins is generally a good rule; however, it is equally important to emphasize that using analgesics more than 2 to 3 days per week can actually begin to increase the frequency and severity of headaches over time. It is important to explain the process of analgesic rebound in simple terms to both parents and children and underscore the importance of parents carefully monitoring their child's analgesic intake.

> **Case Presentation:** A 12-year-old female has episodic migraine controlled well with a prescription combination analgesic. The medication is dispensed in school by a school nurse. After several weeks, the child reports progression to daily headaches. The child and parents are scared about the increasing frequency. The physician interview reveals that the patient began taking medication on a near daily basis, following advice to take the medication at the first onset of

pain. She increased her frequency of use as she began to become more frightened by the increasing frequency of the headaches. Once this pattern was uncovered in the medical interview, the concept of analgesic rebound was explained again in more detail. Given an understandable explanation of the increased frequency of headache, the child's fear decreased. The school nurse was informed of medication limits, the parents monitored medication use more carefully, and the headaches returned to baseline level.

Lifestyle Modifications

In the chaos of adolescent life, it is truly a wonder that headache is not more frequent than it is. Attempting to balance the responsibilities of school, extracurricular activities, and peer relationships, while trying to cope and comply with authority figures of parents and teachers, is often overwhelming for many adolescents. Regulation of these influences through rational modification of lifestyle, although seemingly unrealistic, does play a significant role in reducing headache frequency and severity.

Lifestyle modifications involving sleep schedules, daily activities, eating habits, and diet should be reviewed, and efforts made to effect change. Figures 8–1 and 8–2 are excerpts from the patient information sheet used in our office that emphasize both pharmacologic and nonpharmacologic measures.

Sleep

Either too much, too little, or inconsistent sleep patterns contribute to headache frequency. Particularly during adolescence, deviation from established patterns of sleep can precipitate or exacerbate headache cycles.

Case Presentation: A 16-year-old female with a 2-year history of infrequent migraine headache presents with a daily headache pattern. The headaches are frontal and pounding, are accompanied by photo- and phonophobia, and occur each day about noon. During the calendar school year, she arises at 6 am, catches the bus at 7:15 am, and gets out of school at 4:30 pm following band practice. Since the beginning of summer vacation, she has worked at a fast food restaurant from 4 pm until 11 pm, has gone to bed at midnight, and has

---

What do I do when a headache comes?

If your doctor has given you pain medicine, take it as soon as you feel the pain beginning—Don't wait!!

When a headache attack occurs, try and get to a cool, dark, quiet place and lie down with a cool wash cloth across your forehead. REST!

Sometimes, the doctor may also give you medicine for an upset stomach, if you need it.

If you have learned relaxation techniques, stress relief measures, or biofeedback exercises, begin to use them as soon as the headache starts and before it gets severe.

Figure 8–1   Excerpt from patient education sheet.

arisen at about noon. Her headaches increased 1 week after taking this job. Her examination was normal. Since she has changed shifts to be home by 6 pm and begun to arise at 7 am, her headaches have returned to baseline frequency.

How can I keep the attacks from coming back?

Although there is no 100% sure way to prevent headache attacks, there are lots of effective preventive measures!

First, follow the guidelines for lifestyle changes listed below:
- Eat regularly, do not skip meals.
- Keep a regular sleep schedule.
- Exercise regularly.
- Look for triggers: diet, stress, overexertion, activities.
- Watch for food triggers: cheese, processed meats, chocolates, caffeine, monosodium glutamate, nuts, red wines, pickles …

About one-third of migraine sufferers can identify food triggers.

You don't need to avoid these foods unless one of them triggers off your headache.

We have psychologists available who are skilled in teaching stress management as well as a technique called biofeedback, which can help you take control of your headache.

Your doctor will tailor a program of treatment that may include preventive medications coupled with these psychologic strategies.

Figure 8–2   Excerpt from patient education sheet.

Activities

As part of the comprehensive history, the patient's daily activities should be reviewed. A chronology of daily events will assist with appreciation of the lifestyle and identify provocative or aggravating phenomena. Some overachieving adolescents so completely fill their waking hours that there is no time for self-reflection or relaxation, as shown in the case below.

> **Case Presentation:** A 17-year-old female presents with chronic daily headache. The headaches have been present for 8 months and begin each day about 9 am. The character of the pain varies from squeezing, band-like pain to periodic intense pounding pain. She has maintained a 4.0 grade point average and is vice president of the student council. She is in the Latin Club, thespian troop, honor court, and plays two varsity sports. She is active in her church and teaches Sunday school. She takes 4 to 6 acetaminophen per day. Her examination is normal. She has chronic daily headache with a mixed pattern of milder, frequent tension-type headache and periodic superimposed intense migraine headaches.
>
> This is known as the "valedictorian syndrome": the overachieving adolescent who overextends herself by assuming more and more responsibility at the expense of her own health and well-being. She was carefully advised to scale back her involvement, limit her activities, and begin a program of stress management and biofeedback. Acetaminophen was stopped with concerns of rebound headache. Amitriptyline, 10 mg orally at bedtime each day, was prescribed for prophylaxis. Naproxen sodium (375 mg) was used for moderate headaches and a triptan agent was used for the severe migraine attacks only. Although she is not headache-free, she is much improved.

Conversely, some pediatric patients withdraw from a normal level of activities due to recurrent headache. These patients become more isolated from peers, risk significant developmental delays, and may begin to experience depression. Some parents may even place limits on sports or other normal activities due to concern about possible headache aggravation. Although excessive activity may be a problem, inactivity and withdrawal are equally serious concerns. It is critical for the child or adolescent with recurrent headaches to maintain a normal lifestyle as much as possible. Children and adolescents should continue to participate in regular family activities, such as meals, and maintain certain chores. Withdrawn adolescents may actually benefit from immersing themselves in activities, which may serve as a distraction from their headaches. With frequent and severe headaches, the child and adolescent must learn to set reasonable goals with regard to involvement in activities and then let the goals guide their behavior rather than allow the headache to take control.

Diet

The role of diet and headache is controversial and few studies have documented a clear beneficial effect of dietary elimination schedules. Traditionally, cheeses, processed meats, pickles, monosodium glutamate, and chocolates have been banned from the diets of migraine sufferers, but the reason for doing this is unsubstantiated. The one dietary element that warrants elimination is caffeine because of dependency issues and withdrawal effects.

A reasonable approach is to review the list of foods that have been linked to triggering headache and ask the patient to note any temporal associations between the ingestion of the foods and the development of headache. If an association is uncovered, then common sense would dictate its avoidance; however, wholesale elimination of an arbitrary list of food is not reasonable, and patients will not be comply. Children and adolescents often prefer a rather limited array of foods, and parent-child conflict over foods that are potential, but not clearly demonstrated, headache triggers is not necessarily a good thing.

Exercise

Although there are a small number of outcome studies on the headache-related impact of exercise,[8] we are aware of no controlled studies that demonstrate a decrease in headache frequency or intensity associated with exercise. A review of 10 patient education websites using the search term "headache" discloses the clear recommendation for regular exercise programs for tension-type headache, migraine, and chronic daily headache. In our practices, we routinely encourage regular exercise programs for our patients with frequent headaches. Anecdotally, some patients do report significant headache improvement as their exercise level increases. Of course, vigorous exercise can be a headache trigger, and intensification of head pain during exercise is one of the International Headache Society criteria for migraine. However, most patients can tolerate exercise if the intensity is kept at a moderate level.

Behavioral Therapies

Many allopathic physicians are unfamiliar with (or uncomfortable with) psychologic therapies. They are so vested in the pharmacologic approach to treatment that they often overlook these valuable strategies. As mentioned above, the efficacy of these techniques is well documented and surpasses that of many standard drug regimens. Therefore, it is essential to have access to psychologic services so that treatments such as biofeedback, stress management, relaxation therapy, and cognitive therapies may be used. Before discussing drug treatment plans, it is perfectly reasonable to outline all the available options and then to tailor a regimen to fit the individual patient's profile.

Stress Management

The first step in stress management is identification of the stressors. The most common sources of stress for children or adolescents are marital or family conflict, rejection or hassassment by peers at school, depression, anxiety, sleep disturbances, academic challenges, and sexual, physical, or emotional abuse.[4]

In an outstanding review of behavioral treatments for pediatric headaches, McGrath and Reid recommend maintenance of a headache diary or log in which stressors and medications are recorded and which serves as a way for the child to take control of his or her headache. Stress management entails identification of stressors and reactions to stress, changing thoughts and images about stressful situations, and acquisition of coping techniques to manage stress.[2,4]

Cognitive Therapy

This is a logical follow-up and complement to stress management and essentially involves giving the child insight into the vicious cycle of stress or other triggers and headache.

The first step is the recognition of negative thoughts precipitated by the stressors. Negative thoughts may include elaborate exaggerations, such as "This headache will never go away," or "I can't stop thinking about this headache." Internalization or externalization of blame is another form of negative thought: "It is all my fault," or "The stupid teacher made the exam too hard."

The second step is the process of gaining insight into these negative thoughts and challenging their validity. The counselor will assist the patient in realizing that all past headaches have gone away, so the next one will go away too.

The third cognitive step is to substitute positive thoughts, such as "This is going to be okay," for negative ones or to teach patients to distract themselves so that they think about more pleasant thoughts. This final step must be associated with some reward or self-confidence building statement to reinforce and maintain the positive mood—"I beat this headache again," or "Now I know how to handle this thing."[2,4,9]

Relaxation

Relaxation therapies include progressive muscle relaxation, imagery-based relaxation, and variations of breathing exercises and hybrid forms. Massage therapy and self-hypnosis can also be considered relaxation techniques.

Holden et al. recently critically reviewed the available literature and found 11 studies, which tested the efficacy of relaxation/self-hypnosis/guided imagery as a treatment for childhood headache. Although the results are mixed and the study populations heterogeneous, the authors concluded that sufficient evidence exists that relaxation/self-hypnosis is a well-established and efficacious treatment for recurrent migraine and tension-type headache in children.[2]

Massage.   Massaging tense muscles can be quite relaxing and comforting not only to prevent headache but also to treat attacks of headache. Massage may be self-performed or performed by a parent or massage therapist and viewed within the context of relaxation programs.

Hypnosis.   Two studies have documented the efficacy of hypnosis for pediatric headache.[10,11] Hypnosis is a blend of relaxation, imagery, and the power of suggestion to achieve a heightened sense of relaxation. Hypnosis therapists use a variety of techniques such as hand levitation, eye closure, and guided imagery. Headache relief is achieved through deep relaxation and posthypnotic suggestion.[10]

Olness et al. compared self-hypnosis with propranolol for treating juvenile migraine in a prospective fashion and found a statistically significant reduction in headache frequency in the self-hypnosis group but little change in headache severity.[12]

Biofeedback

The mechanism underlying the therapeutic benefits of biofeedback is poorly understood. Nonetheless, a growing body of literature has evolved using various forms of biofeedback including cephalic vasomotor biofeedback, electromyographic biofeedback, relaxation training, cognitive coping skills training, contingency management, and skin temperature feedback with autogenic training, all of which have been used in childhood headache. Of these interventions, skin temperature biofeedback with autogenic training has received the majority of recent attention and beneficial reports.[13]

In a recent review by Holden et al., 17 studies of the usefulness of biofeedback were analyzed. Seven of the studies specifically assessed biofeedback, whereas 10 investigations used biofeedback as part of a multimodal or combined strategy with self-hypnosis and relaxation programs. The authors believe that enough evidence exists to conclude that thermal biofeedback alone is "probably efficacious" treatment for childhood headache but is arguably a "well-established treatment" for pediatric migraine. Furthermore, the combined biofeedback and relaxation/self-hypnosis were viewed as "promising" but methodologically inadequate to make clear efficacy determinations.[2]

The process of thermal biofeedback involves 45-minute sessions wherein during the first 15 minutes the patient sits quietly to establish a baseline skin temperature. The next 15 minutes consist of skin temperature biofeedback, and the final 15 minutes consist of self-control of skin temperature. The thermal biofeedback is performed by using a temperature thermistor and monitored from the volar surface of the distal phalanges.[2,4,13,14] These techniques are first learned in the office setting then practiced at home, eventually being used during the course of everyday activities. Success rates, as measured by decreased headache severity and frequency, of up to 80% are reported.[13]

Although it has been customary to use skin temperature biofeedback for migraine headache and muscle biofeedback for tension-type headache, McGrath and Reid point out that there are no convincing data suggesting such specificity of treatment modalities and that it is likely that most children could benefit from both forms of biofeedback.[4] There are little data to suggest one technique is more superior to the other, but combining relaxation with other modalities, such as biofeedback, may improve overall effectiveness.

As with any type of relaxation therapy or biofeedback training, practice is important. Parents need to express interest and may participate in the process with younger children. The physician and other treating professionals should ask about the frequency of practice and provide ongoing reinforcement and encouragement.

Addressing School Issues

School is a commonly identified stressor for children with headache and can be blamed for triggering headaches.[1] School problems were identified in 46% of patients between ages 5 and 17 in a pediatric practice and were more common than vomiting, dizziness, or neurologic accompaniments.[15] The child's history must be probed to determine if the child is being teased or bullied by classmates or if there may be occult learning disabilities as the source of the headache. Headache can affect the child's ability to concentrate in class and when doing homework.[16] Almost 2 out of 5 children with migraine (37%) report that they perform poorly during headache.[17] Fear of failure and school problems have been significantly correlated with headache, especially in higher grades.[18]

When headache is frequent and intractable, school attendance and school-related behavior can cause great child and parental distress and must be directly addressed in treatment. The National Health Interview Survey revealed that headache ranks third among illness-related causes of school absence.[19] However, it is a minority of intractable pediatric headache patients with frequent and severe headaches who accounts for the majority of school days lost, with 10% of this group missing at least 2 days of school per month, and 1% missing 2 or more days of school per week.[20] In some cases, headache may be most prevalent on school days, with minimal problems on weekends or school vacations.

Underlying issues interfering with school attendance can include fear of pain, headache-related reading and performance problems, difficulty coping with headache-related academic impairment, and undiagnosed learning disabilities. Some headache sufferers experience or fear harassment from other students and even teachers on occasion. Parental issues can range from reinforcement of pain behavior at home to difficulty monitoring attendance due to work schedules, parental distress, and strongly held beliefs about the perceived cruelty of sending a child with pain to school. In addition, there may be conflict between the parents over whether the child should attend school with a severe headache.

In some cases, behavioral contracts specifying a school attendance plan and reinforcement contingencies for compliance can be very helpful. Therapeutic effort must often focus on helping parents understand the importance of helping their child function in the presence of pain to the fullest extent possible to maintain developmental progress and minimize future disability. Communication and cooperation between the treatment providers and the school is essential, particularly since some schools are under state or board requirements regarding minimal levels of acceptable attendance even when illness is a factor. In some cases, a graduated return to school beginning with 1 to 2 hours per day, regardless of headache level, can create a foundation for eventual full-time attendance. In others, the contract may need to insist on full time attendance as a requirement for continuing treatment.

Case Presentation: A 13-year-old girl who has intractable migraine with aura and comorbid insulin-dependent diabetes failed to show any sustained improvement with over 18 months of treatment, including biofeedback, individual psychotherapy, family therapy, intensive pharmacotherapy, and two hospitalizations. Although regular school attendance had been repeatedly emphasized as a critical component of successful treatment, she continued to miss several days of school a week despite agreement to attend. Finally, her treating doctor informed the family that he would no longer continue to treat her unless she began full-time attendance, regardless of pain. The school provided a quiet area to which she could retreat if necessary. It was only when the continued relationship with the physician was made contingent on regular attendance that she actually began to attend school consistently. Her headaches gradually began to improve, and her fear of handling headaches in the school setting waned as she confronted the situation. She caught up academically with her classmates. Although at first she was very unhappy about the school attendance demand, both she and her parents came to recognize this as a key factor in her improvement.

One word of caution: consider homebound programs only as a last resort! If a well-meaning clinician permits the child or adolescent to gain a home-bound program after identifying the school as a trigger, a very difficult situation invariably arises when determining the length of home stay or when attempting to get the child back into school. The child will very strongly resist any effort to restore him or her to school, and the parents will become wrapped up in this battle. The child must eventually be returned to the mainstream of life, which for a teenager is school, and this will not be an easy process.

Individual and Family Therapy

Chronic headache in children and adolescents increases the risk of psychiatric comorbidity. In one long-term epidemiologic study of children between the ages of 9 and 18, 24% of those with headache sufficient to cause functional impairment (10% of the population) also met criteria for major depression within 7 years.[21] Headache was about twice as common in depressed versus nondepressed adolescents. Conversely, the presence of multiple psychiatric disorders lends an unfavorable prognosis for headache outcome. An 8-year follow-up of 100 adolescents and young adults found that for those with more than one psychiatric disorder, 57% were the same or worse compared with only 15% of those with one disorder and 7% of those with no psychiatric comorbidity.[22] The clinician needs to be attuned to the possibility of comorbid psychiatric complications in the refractory patient. Although there is no good evidence supporting psychotherapy as a lone treatment for pediatric headache, it can be an important part of an overall treatment program for a significant number of patients.

The amount of parental distress displayed in front of the child is significantly related to the amount of distress shown by children undergoing routine medical procedures,[23] and may also affect a child's distress in response to recurrent, painful conditions, such as chronic headache. Significant correlations have been found between the amount of parent negativity and headache-related behavior problems in adolescents. More affiliative, affectionate parental behavior is associated with less headache-related functional disability in younger children.[24] Problems between the parents have been associated with headache in children and adolescents,[25] although the quality of family relationships appears unrelated to outcome from behavioral treatment.[26] Sometimes parents provide too much attention or reinforcement of pain behavior and fail to encourage and reinforce functioning when the child feels uncomfortable. Treating professionals should open discussion of these issues, particularly if the child or adolescent is not showing evidence of improvement. Family therapy that addresses these concerns can be the key to treatment success in some intractable cases.

CONCLUSION

The purpose of this chapter was to outline available nonpharmacologic treatments for pediatric headache. Confident reassurance is our most valuable initial therapeutic intervention. Once physicians have adequately convinced themselves of the nature of the headache, patients and their families can be relieved of the burden of fear by a clear statement that the headache is not being caused by a life-threatening disease.

When formulating a treatment strategy, both pharmacologic and psychologic measures should be considered. Again, the value of many of the nonpharmacologic strategies has been well validated by controlled series perhaps as well as or even better than some of the traditional pharmacologic agents discussed in Chapter 6.

The prudent clinician will not discount the potentially beneficial effects of nonpharmacologic management and will make efforts to identify sources in their community who are skilled in these therapeutic options. The most frequently employed techniques include stress management, cognitive therapy, relaxation techniques, and biofeedback. A combined program of relaxation training, stress management, and thermal biofeedback has received the most clinical and research attention and rationally takes advantage of multiple psychologic strategies toward the effort of decreasing headache frequency and severity.

REFERENCES

1. Lewis DW, Middlebrook MT, Mehallick L, et al. Pediatric headaches: what do the children want? Headache 1996;36:224–230.
2. Holden EW, Deichmann MM, Levy JD. Empirically supported treatments in pediatric psychology: recurrent pediatric headache. J Pediatr Psychol 1999;24:91–109.
3. Herman C, Kim M, Blanchard ED. Behavioral and prophylactic pharmacological intervention studies of pediatric migraine: and exploratory meta-analysis. Pain 1995;60:239–256.
4. McGrath PJ, Reid GJ. Behavioral treatment of pediatric headache. Pediatr Ann 1995;24:486–491.
5. Sartory G, Muller B, Mecsch J, et al. A comparison of psychological and pharmacological treatment of pediatric migraine. Behav Res Ther 1998; 36:1155–1170.
6. Jensen VK, Rothner AD. Chronic nonprogressive headache in children and adolescents. Semin Pediatr Neurol 1995;2:151–158.
7. Mathews N, Kurman R, Perez F. Drug induced refractory headache—clinical features and management. Headache 1990;30:634–638.
8. Peters M, Turner S, Blanchard E. The effects of aerobic exercise on chronic tension-type headache. Headache 1996;7(4):330–344.
9. Womack WM, Smith MS, Chen ACN. Behavioral management of childhood headache: a pilot study and case history report. Pain 1988;32:279–283.
10. Kapelis L. Hypnosis in a behaviour therapy framework for the treatment of headache in children. Aust J Clin Exp Hypn 1984;12:123–126.
11. Smith MS, Womack WM, Chen AC. Hypnotizability does not predict outcome of behavioral treatment in pediatric headache. Am J Clin Hypn 1989;31:237–241.
12. Olness K, MacDonald JT, Uden DL. Comparison of self-hypnosis and propranolol in the treatment of juvenile classic migraine. Pediatrics 1987; 79:593–597.
13. Labbe EE. Treatment of childhood migraine with autogenic training and skin temperature biofeedback: a component analysis. Headache 1994;35:10–13.

14. Allen KD, Shriver MD. Enhanced performance feedback to strengthen biofeedback treatment outcome in childhood migraine. Headache 1997; 37:169–173.

15. Nealis JG, Miller S. School problems and other factors in childhood headache syndromes. J Learn Disabil 1984;17:556–559.

16. King NJ, Sharpley CF. Headache activity in children and adolescents. J Paediatr Child Health 1990:26:50–54.

17. Lee LH, Olness KN. Clinical and demographic characteristics of migraine in urban children. Headache 1997;37:269–276.

18. Alfven G. The covariation of common psychosomatic symptoms among children from socio-economically differing residential areas. An epidemiological study. Acta Pediatr 1993;82:484–487.

19. Newacheck PW, Taylor WR. Childhood chronic illness: prevalence, severity, and impact. Am J Public Health 1992:82:364–371.

20. Stang PE, Osterhouse JT. Impact of migraine in the United States: data from the National Health Interview Survey. Headache 1993;33:29–35.

21. Pine DS, Cohen P, Brook J. The association between major depression and headache: results of a longitudinal epidemiologic study in youth. J Child Adolesc Psychopharmacol 1996;6:153–164.

22. Guidetti V, Galli F, Fabrizi P, et al. Headache and psychiatric comorbidity: clinical aspects and outcome in an 8-year follow-up study. Cephalalgia 1998;18:455–462.

23. Frank NC, Blount RL, Smith AJ, et al. Parent and staff behavior, previous child medical experience, and maternal anxiety as they relate to child procedural distress and coping. J Pediatr Psychol 1994;20:277–289.

24. Wall BA, Holden EW, Gladstein J. Parent responses to pediatric headache. Headache 1997;37:65–70.

25. Metsahonkala L, Sillanpaa M, Tuominen J. Outcome of early school age migraine. Cephalalgia 1997;17:662–665.

26. Hermann C, Blanchard EB, Flor H. Biofeedback treatment for pediatric migraine: prediction of treatment outcome. J Consult Clin Psychol 1997; 65:531–541.

Chapter 9

POST-TRAUMATIC HEADACHE

Paul Winner and
Stephen D. Silberstein

Children and adolescents who are involved in motor vehicle accidents, bicycle accidents, sports-related injuries, or child abuse may develop a headache syndrome within 24 hours to weeks following the incident, even after what would seem to be a trivial head injury. Most children who are hospitalized following a head injury have a Glasgow coma scale between 13 and 15 (Table 9–1). Patients who have Glasgow coma scales of less than 8 account for approximately 5% of hospital admissions. Headaches that occur following a minor head injury often clear within

Table 9–1 Glasgow Coma Scale	
Eye opening	
Spontaneous	4
To sound	3
To pain	2
None	1
Verbal response	
Oriented	5
Confused	4
Inappropriate	3
Incomprehensible	2
None	1
Best motor response	
Obeys	6
Localizes	5
Withdraws	4
Abnormal flexion	3
Extends	2
None	1

2 to 3 months. Headache and the constellation of symptoms that occur following trauma are sometimes referred to as post-traumatic or postconcussion syndrome. The associated symptoms include vertigo, dizziness, difficulty concentrating, memory disorders, depression, altered school performance, behavior disorders, and sleep alteration.[1-3] The pathophysiology of post-traumatic headache and postconcussion syndrome following minor head injuries is not as well understood as that which occurs following a severe head injury. The severity of the symptoms does not depend on the severity of the head injury. Severe headaches, impaired memory, and difficulty concentrating have been reported with both traumatic and relatively minor head injuries.[4] The headaches associated with the postconcussion syndrome can be similar to a migraine headache, a tension-type headache, or both, and are often referred to as chronic daily or mixed headache. Cluster-type headaches have even been reported following a head injury.[5] Children without concussion symptoms and mild head injury Glasgow coma scales of 13 to 15 may have symptoms ranging from no detectable structural abnormality to focal periangular brain lesions or dural hemorrhages.

The clinical and neurobehavioral abnormalities following mild head injury have been fairly well established using a monkey model for a minor acceleration/deceleration nonimpact head injury in the sagittal plane where the animal sustained a brief loss of consciousness but no reported neurologic deficits.[6] Degenerating axons were noted in the pons and dorsal midbrain 7 days postinjury. Injuries in experimental animals and humans suggest that trauma causes a disorganization of the neurofilament cytoskeleton and axolemma and results in axonal disconnection.[7] A minor acceleration/deceleration injury that involves rotational forces may result in axonal shearing or tearing, especially in areas of the midbrain, superior cerebellar peduncles, corpus callosum, and central white matter of the brain.[8] Acceleration/deceleration of the brain may also damage the labyrinth and mechanoreceptor in the neck and central vestibular connections, resulting in the symptoms of dizziness and vertigo that are often reported by patients with postconcussion syndrome. Blood vessels may be stretched or injured during the head injury; this impairs the vascular contractility in autoregulation that may result from direct vascular damage or may be a residual from tissue injury. Acceleration/deceleration forces may also result in stretch and strain of the cervical ligaments and muscles and the supporting bony structures of the neck and back.[9] Postconcussion syndrome symptoms are more common after a mild to moderate head injury than after a severe head injury. Direct impact is not necessary for postconcussion syndrome.[10] The unsynchronized rotational forces that may develop between the cerebral hemisphere in the cerebellum and the axons in the upper brain stem are more vulnerable to diffuse axonal injury; this may play a role in explaining the symptom complex that develops following head injury. The persistence of headache and associated symptoms may not correlate with the duration of unconsciousness, post-traumatic amnesia, or skull fracture. Clearly further work is necessary to understand the pathophysiology and clinical relationship of this information. A concussion produced by rotational forces to a semisolid brain within a skull can give rise to shearing and diffuse axonal injury.[7] This correlation with clinical symptomatology needs to be addressed further.

DIAGNOSIS

As we gain a greater understanding of neurophysiology, our understanding of the pathophysiology of head pain and its associated symptom complex will occur (Table 9–2). The guidelines established by the International Headache Society require that headache onset occurs within 2 weeks of the head injury or from the time the patient regains consciousness to be considered a post-traumatic injury. This appears to be a reasonable guide, although patients report headache onset as long as 1 month after the injury. This may be due to the fact that other injuries were sustained or other symptoms were more distressing.

Some patients report migraine-like headaches following the injury; however, they often do not respond well to standard migraine medications.[11–13] The neurologic sequelae of mild head injuries in children and adolescents who report headache include hyperactivity, difficulty concentrating, memory disorders, vertigo, dizziness, depression, and altered personality causing altered school performance and behavior disorders (Table 9–3).[14,15] Both the patient and the family must be assured that the associated symptoms are common but will probably resolve over the next several weeks to months and that most children will be symptom-free within a few months.

Table 9–2   Post-traumatic Headache

Begins in days or weeks
Migraine-like quality
Cognitive difficulties
Symptoms may not equal injury
Subsides spontaneously?

Patients under the age of 12 years who have a sports-related injury rarely sustain a severe brain injury.[16] The potential for long-term sequelae following minor head injury in young athletes is unknown. There is concern regarding second impact syndrome. In this situation, a young athlete with a minor head injury recovers uneventfully; however, if the child sustains another minor head injury sometime within the next week, rapid cerebral edema occurs and death follows.[17] There may be compound effects of sequential minor injuries to the brain with resultant cerebral swelling and diminished intracranial compliance. Thus, the issue of when an athlete can return to play following a minor head injury is controversial and new guidelines have been proposed.[18]

Headaches in children may be caused by idiopathic intracranial hypertension, pseudotumor cerebri with or without papilledema, minor head injury, carotid sheath injury, and temporomandibular injury. Temporomandibular disorder may be a headache trigger.[19] Some children report sleep disturbances, including insomnia, daytime drowsiness, nonspecific staring episodes, periodic loss of consciousness, neurocognitive deficits, and an inability to process information.[20]

Table 9–3   Postconcussion Syndrome Following Minor Head Injury

Headache
Hyperactivity
Decreased attention span
Sleep disturbances
Behavior disorders
Dizziness

Adapted from: Rizzo M, Tranel D. Head Injury and Post Concussive Syndrome. New York: Churchill Livingston, 1996, p 449.

DIAGNOSTIC EVALUATIONS

Most patients who are hospitalized for a mild to moderate head injury receive some form of neuroimaging — either computed tomography (CT) or magnetic resonance imaging (MRI). The absence of abnormality on MRI or CT does not predict whether a patient will develop post-traumatic headaches or postconcussion syndrome. Patients who have a mild behavior abnormality and a Glasgow coma scale of less than 15 should have an MRI of the brain to rule out chronic subdural hematoma, hydrocephalus, or a structural lesion unrelated to the trauma.[21] If a patient has associated cervical symptoms, an MRI of the cervical region should be obtained. In the future, single photon emission computed tomography (SPECT) may prove to be a beneficial instrument. Initial studies suggest that this form of imaging may be helpful in predicting central nervous system (CNS) outcomes.[22–24] Early assessments indicate that SPECT scans may be somewhat more sensitive as long-term outcome predictors than CT or MRI scans.[25]

Brain stem auditory–evoked potentials have been found to be abnormal in 10 to 20% of individuals with head injury-associated postconcussion syndrome.[21] This relationship and its usefulness as a predictor for postconcussion sequelae need further assessment.

NEUROPSYCHOLOGIC TESTING

In patients with postconcussion syndrome, abnormalities may be found in information processing, auditory vigilance, reaction time, attention, visual and verbal memory, and analytic capacity.[26] Following mild head injury, there seems to be a hierarchy of functional recovery in those individuals who do recover, which is the vast majority of children and adolescents. Attention and concentration deficits usually resolve within 6 weeks. Visual memory, imagination, and analytic capacity also resolve but not for 6 weeks. Verbal memory, abstraction, cognitive selectivity, and information processing speed may take more than 12 weeks to recover.[26]

Migraine, tension-type, cluster, and chronic daily cluster headache patterns have all been reported in patients with minor head injury.[27,28] Patients who reported post-traumatic headache commonly had a prior history of headache.[29,30] Although many children have clinical improvement of their headache sequelae within several weeks, and most within several months, some patients never have complete recovery with regard to headache and the associated symptoms of postconcussion syndrome. Adult patients have been reported to have continuing symptoms for 3 to 5 years after the injury that are independent of financial compensation.[31-33] The formal diagnosis of post-traumatic headaches and postconcussion syndrome requires that the constellation of symptoms is present and its onset is related to the trauma. Subdural hemorrhage, cerebral vein thrombosis, cavernous sinus thrombosis, carotid artery dissection, epilepsy, cerebral hemorrhage, CNS neoplasm, and hydrocephalus must be ruled out.[21] Head injury accounts for the largest number of emergency department visits by children.[34]

TREATMENT

Managing children and adolescents with head injury requires rapid clinical assessment, as well as anticipation of the potential for intracranial complications. Post-traumatic headache treatment is symptomatic. Patients with post-traumatic headaches are often misdiagnosed or undiagnosed, and parents of children and adolescents may dismiss the complaints as being "only a headache." The issue may be further complicated if other associated symptoms of postconcussion syndrome are present and undiagnosed or not related to the recent head injury. Thus, the most beneficial approach is to educate the parents and the patient as to what potentially may occur. Simply discussing what post-traumatic headache and postconcussion syndrome are and what may occur in the next several weeks and months may be therapeutic.

The initial headache symptoms and soft tissue injuries may be effectively treated with mild analgesics and nonsteroidal anti-inflammatory drugs (NSAIDs) over the initial several weeks. If there are associated cervical soft tissue symptoms, a short course of physical therapy might be of benefit, depending on the patient's age and circumstances. If more prominent headache symptomatology or associated symptoms of anxiety, depression, or cognitive difficulties are present, more aggressive intervention may be necessary.

Post-traumatic headache usually responds to the medications that are used for chronic daily headache and chronic tension-type headache, although no specific medication or treatment protocol has been found that will alter the underlying CNS disturbance, nor is there a clearly defined treatment protocol. Tricyclic antidepressants, such as amitriptyline (Elavil) or nortriptyline (Pamelor) are often the medications of choice. In children, the cardiac side effects are of concern. The β-blockers may also prove helpful, although these drugs may potentiate fatigue or produce depression. Cyproheptadine, a drug that produces sedation, may be helpful, especially for patients with sleep disorders, since it can be given as a single night-time dose. If patients are having frequent headaches, it is important to talk about medication overuse or the possibility of developing rebound headaches. Analgesic use should be limited to no more than twice a week. The NSAID use should be limited to two to three times a week since these drugs have the potential to cause rebound headaches. The NSAIDs have potential gastrointentinal and renal side effects in this population and need to be carefully monitored if they are to be used long term.

Patients who have migraine-like post-traumatic headaches may benefit from triptans, with or without antiemetics. Some patients may respond to dihydroergotamine (D.H.E. 45), especially if there is a persistent, refractory headache pattern. Nonpharmacologic therapies, such as biofeedback and stress management techniques, can be quite effective, even in children as young as 9 years of age.[14] It is important that teachers and other family members be aware of postconcussion syndrome and its potential sequelae, especially when children are having difficulty in school following a minor head injury. A psychologist may be helpful for teaching coping mechanisms for pain to older children and adolescents. If symptoms do not resolve in several weeks or a few months, physiologic testing should be considered and medication regimens reassessed.[35]

It was believed that young children are less vulnerable to long-term sequelae of brain injury than older children or adults. Recent research does not support the concept that younger brains recover better or more comprehensively after injury.[36] Differences based on focal lesions are not consistently seen, and younger brains do not appear to recover better than those of older children or adults.[37–39] The relationship between age and CNS injury outcome is quite complex and depends on a variety of factors involving the nature and timing of the injury and the environmental contacts.[40] It is believed that skills that are undergoing development are more vulnerable to CNS or cerebral injury than well-formulated skills.[41] Present evidence suggests that outcomes following minor head injuries are similar in adults and children.[42,43]

Since different definitions of head injury and different study designs have been used, it is difficult to ascertain the prognosis of post-traumatic headache in the studies available. One month after mild head injury, up to 90% of adult patients reported headache;[44] 2 to 3 months postinjury, up to 78% reported headache.[15] One year post–head injury, 35 to 54% of patients reported headache symptoms.[45] Two to 4 years after injury, 20 to 24% of patients reported persistent headache symptomatology. Approximately one-third of adults are unable to return to work after a head injury.[46]

There are no precise criteria for predicting the clinical outcome of children and adolescents following head injury. Headache gradually improves over a period of 3 to 6 months. Children who experience persistent symptoms that do not abate over the course of months to years are believed to have sustained a diffuse injury resulting from acceleration/deceleration forces. Children and adolescents may benefit from a combination of pharmacologic and nonpharmacologic therapies for symptomatic relief. Patients who do not fully recover within 6 months after injury may benefit from neurophysiologic testing to formulate recommendations for future intervention, although earlier assessments may prove beneficial for those children who have more significant difficulties even a few months after a minor head injury.

ACKNOWLEDGMENT

We appreciate the assistance of Lynne Kaiser with the completion of this chapter.

REFERENCES

1. Evans RW. The postconcussion syndrome and the sequelae of mild head injury. Neurol Clin 1992;10:815–847.
2. Rizzo M, Tranel D. Pediatric Trauma. Eichelberge: Mosby, 1993, pp 352–361.
3. Goldstein B, Powers KS. Head trauma in children. Pediatr Rev 1994;15:213–219.

4. Rizzo M, Tranel D. Head Injury and Post Concussive Syndrome. New York: Churchill Livingston, 1996, pp 51–52.

5. Reik L. Cluster headache after head injury. Headache 1987;27:509–510.

6. Jane JA, Steward O, Gennarelli T. Axonal degeneration induced by experimental noninvasive minor head injury. J Neurosurg 1985;62:96–100.

7. Christman CW, Grady MS, Walker SA, et al. Ultrastructural studies of diffuse axonal injury in humans. J Neurotrauma 1994;11:173–186.

8. Rizzo M, Tranel D. Head Injury and Post Concussive Syndrome. New York: Churchill Livingston, 1996, p 55.

9. Gordon B. Postconcussional syndrome. In: Johnson RT, editor. Current Therapy in Neurologic Disease. Philadelphia: B C Decker, 1990, pp 208–213.

10. Gennarelli TA. Mechanisms of brain injury. J Emerg Med 1993;1:511.

11. Evans RW. The postconcussion syndrome and the sequelae of mild head injury. Neurol Clin 1992;10:815–847.

12. Mandel S. Minor head injury may not be "minor." Postgrad Med 1989;85: 213–215.

13. Brenner C, Friendman AP, Merritt HH, et al. Post-traumatic headache. J Neurosurg 1944;1:317–391.

14. Winner P. Post-traumatic headache. In: Maria BL. Current Management in Child Neurology. Hamilton, ON: B C Decker, 1999, pp 57–58.

15. Rimel RW, Giordani B, Barth JT, et al. Disability caused by minor head injury. Neurosurgery 1981;9(3):221–228.

16. Bruce DA, Schut L, Sutton LN. Brain and cervical spine injuries occurring during organized sports activities in children and adolescents. Clin Sports Med 1982;1:495–514.

17. Saudners RL, Harbaugh RE. The second impact in catastrophic contact-sports head trauma. JAMA 1984;252:538–539.

18. Rizzo M, Tranel D. Head Injury and Post Concussive Syndrome. New York: Churchill Livingston, 1996, p 449.

19. Silberstein S, Marceils J. Pseudotumor cerebri without papilledema. Headache 1990;30:304.

20. Gronwall D, Wrightston P. Delayed recovery of intellectual function after minor head injury. Lancet 1974;2:605–609.

21. Silberstein S, Lipton R, Goadsby P. Post-traumatic headache. In: Silberstein S, Lipton R, Goadsby P, eds. Headache in Clinical Practice. Corby, UK: Oxford University Press, 1998, p 139.

22. Abdel-Dayem HM, Sadek SA, Kouris K, et al. Changes in cerebral perfusion after acute head injury: comparison of CT with Tc: 99m – PAO SPECT. Radiology 1987;165:221–226.

23. Reid, RH, Gulenchyn KY, Ballinger JR, Ventureyra EC. Cerebral perfusion imaging with technetium-99m HMPAO following cerebral trauma. Initial experience. Clin Nucl Med 1990;15:383–388.

24. Abdel-Dayem H, Masdeu J, O'Connel R, et al. Brain perfusion abnormalities following minor/moderate closed head injury: comparison between early and late imaging in two groups of patients. Eur J Nucl Med 1994;21:750.

25. Gray BG, Ichise M, Chung D, et al. Technetium 99-m HMPAO SPECT in the evaluation of patient with a remote history of traumatic brain injury: a comparison with X-ray computed tomography. J Nucl Med 1992;33:52–58.

26. Silberstein S, Lipton R, Goadsby P. Post-traumatic headache. In: Silberstein S, Lipton R, Goadsby P, eds. Headache in Clinical Practice. Corby, UK: Oxford University Press, 1998, pp 140.

27. Weiss HD, Sterm BJ, Goldbert J. Post traumatic migraine: chronic migraine precipitated by minor head or neck trauma. Headache 1991;31:451–456.

28. Haas DC, Laurie H. Trauma-triggered migraine: an explanation for common neurologic attacks after mild head injury. J Neurosurg 1988;68:181–188.

29. Jensen OK, Nielsen FF. The influence of sex and pretraumatic headache on the incidence and severity of headache after head injury. Cephalalgia 1990;10:285–293.

30. Russell MB, Olesen J. Migraine associated with head trauma and its relation to migraine. Eur J Neurol 1996;3:424–428.

31. Medina JL. Efficacy of an individualized outpatient program in the treatment of chronic post-traumatic headache. Headache 1992;32:180–183.

32. Packard RC, Ham LP. Post-traumatic headache: determining chronicity. Headache 1993;33:133–134.

33. Packard RC. Post-traumatic headache: permanency and relationship to legal settlement. Headache 1992;32:496–450.

34. Kraus JF, Fife D, Cox P, et al. Incidence, severity and external causes of pediatric brain injury. Am J Dis Child 1986;140:687–693.

35. Silberstein S, Lipton R, Goadsby P. Post-traumatic headache. In: Silberstein S, Lipton R, Goadsby P, eds. Headache in Clinical Practice. Corby, UK: Oxford University Press, 1998, p 137.

36. Goldman PS. An alternative to development plasticity: heterology of CNS structures in infants and adults. In: Stein DG, Rosen JJ, Butters N, eds. Plasticity and Recovery from Brain Damage. Orlando: Academic Press, 1974, pp 149–174.

37. Mahoney WJ, D'Souza BJ, Haller JA, et al. Long-term outcome of children with severe head trauma and prolonged coma. Pediatrics 1983;71:756–762.

38. Kriel RL, Krach LE, Panser LA. Closed head injury: comparison of children younger and older than 6 years of age. Pediatr Neurol 1989;5:296–300.

39. Filley CM, Cranberg ID, Alexander MP, Hart EJ. Neurobehavioral outcome after closed head injury in childhood and adolescence. Arch Neurol 1987;44:194–198.

40. Kolb B. Brain development, plasticity, and behavior. Am Psychol 1989;44: 1203–1212.

41. Ewing-Cobbs L, Levin HS, Eisenberg HM, Fletcher JM. Language functions following closed-head injury in children and adolescents. J Clin Exp Neuropsychol 1987;9:575–592.

42. Dikman S, McLean A, Temkin N. Neuropsychological and psychosocial consequences of minor head injury. J Neurol Neurosurg Psychiatry 1986;49: 1227–1232.

43. Fay GC, Jaffe KM, Polissar NL, et al. Mild pediatric traumatic brain injury: a cohort study. Arch Phys Med Rehabil 1993;74:895–901.

44. Denker PG. The postconcussion syndrome: prognosis and evaluation of the organic factors. N Y State J Med 1944;44:379–384.

45. Dencker SJ, Lofving BA. A psychometric study of identical twins discordant for closed head injury. Acta Psychiatr Neurol Scand 1968;(Suppl 33): 1958.

46. Rutherford WH, Merrett JD, McDonald JR. Sequelae of concussion caused by minor head injuries. Lancet 1977;1:14.

MISCELLANEOUS
HEADACHE SYNDROMES

A. David Rothner

In this chapter we will review several headache syndromes that do not easily fall into the usual classifications. The majority of these headaches are not associated with structural brain disease and they are less common than the ones previously described. It is important to note, however, that proper identification of these syndromes may lead to specific treatment resulting in dramatic relief of symptoms.

CLUSTER HEADACHES

The character of cluster headaches was first described by Ekbom in 1947.[1] Further delineation of this syndrome by Kunkle et al. in 1952 solidified this as a specific headache syndrome.[2] Two forms of cluster headache occur: chronic and episodic.[3] The chronic form never remits. The episodic is defined by periods of 1 to 3 months during which the headaches are frequent, then by periods of remission, which last months to years. Episodic cluster affects 80% of cluster headache sufferers. In 20% of patients with cluster headache, however, chronic cluster headache occurs. This is the occurrence of cluster headaches without remission. Cluster headaches primarily affect males and the mean onset is in the third decade of life. In a study by Ekbom et al. it was noted that 1% of 18-year-old Swedish men had this disorder.[4] The typical attack occurs from 2 to 10 times daily and lasts 10 minutes to 3 hours, although usually it lasts 45 minutes. It may occur during sleep and awaken the patient during the first phase of rapid eye movement sleep. The intensity of the pain is severe. The location is always unilateral and it almost never changes sides. It is usually localized in or about the eye and is associated with ipsilateral lacrimation, rhinorrhea, and nasal stuffiness. Ipsilateral ptosis and miosis may occur.

Most patients will find it impossible to lie down or rest during a cluster attack. The attacks may be provoked by alcohol, especially during the period when the cluster headaches are active. The differential diagnosis is limited. The disorder is not familial and the pathophysiology is not clear. It is known that histamine can precipitate an attack. Acutely, patients may benefit from oxygen or ergotamine tartrate. Chronically, prophylactic medications have included methysergide, verapamil, lithium, and prednisone.[3]

Cluster headaches are rare in childhood. Maytal et al. identified seven patients with onset prior to age 10.[5] They concluded that cluster headaches in childhood closely resemble the adult forms of the disease.

TEMPOROMANDIBULAR JOINT DISORDER

Children with temporomandibular joint (TMJ) disorders usually present with unilateral pain of a dull aching nature just below the ear in the preauricular area.[6] The pain may remain localized, or it may radiate to the temporal region, toward the middle of the face, or into the frontal region of the skull. The pain is frequently aggravated by chewing. Patients frequently describe clicking and locking of their jaw. The incidence of this disorder in pediatric and adolescent patients is unknown. In clinical practice, this is an uncommon cause of headache.

On examination, there may be no abnormalities noted. Patients, however, may have tenderness over their jaw(s), and there may be palpable slipping of the joint on jaw opening, and actual limitation of mouth opening. The majority of patients have no radiographic abnormality.

The TMJ disorder rarely causes severe pain. It may be caused by rheumatoid arthritis or seen after fractures in that region. More commonly, however, the syndrome is due to excessive muscle spasm and fatigue that may be associated with malocclusion, bruxism, teeth clenching, excessive gum chewing, and stress.

Pillemer et al. in 1987 discussed the entity of TMJ disorder and facial pain as being, in many cases, secondary to reactive depression.[7] In the absence of organic or anatomic TMJ pathology, they felt that a combined approach using anti-inflammatory drugs, muscle relaxants, occlusal splints, biofeedback, counseling, and psychopharmacologic medication is the best approach to this disorder. It is important to emphasize that major dental surgery and costly therapeutic programs should be avoided and are unnecessary in the vast majority of children and adolescents presenting with this form of pain.

OCCIPITAL NEURALGIA

The term "occipital neuralgia" includes pain experienced in the posterior part of the head often starting at the upper neck or base of the skull.[8] It may be unilateral or bilateral. The frequency of the pain ranges anywhere from infrequent pain, to several discrete episodes per day, to continuous pain. The pain is frequently described as jabbing or throbbing and may be seen acutely or chronically. Associated symptoms may include dizziness and, only rarely, nausea or vomiting. The actual pain may radiate frontally or to the eye. Patients, in addition, may report that their scalp seems sensitive to touch. At times, the pain can be brought on by movement, especially extension of the head posteriorly. Physical examination is usually normal. There may, however, be cervical tenderness, limitation of motion, head tilt, and on careful examination, decreased sensation over the C2 dermatome. Patients may be tender to palpation where the nerve crosses the superior nuchal line.

In the paper by Dugan et al. radiographic studies demonstrated abnormalities in the craniovertebral junction and the cervical vertebrae in a number of patients.[9] Athletics, including weight lifting, wrestling, and football, seem to be a precipitating and/or aggravating feature in a number of adolescents whom we have seen.[10] Extension/flexion injuries, as in automobile accidents, can also be causative. Magnetic resonance imaging of the head and neck, with emphasis of the cervicocranial junction, can be helpful. Treatment modalities vary, depending on the severity and acuity of the problem, and include soft cervical collar, analgesics, muscle relaxants, local injections, and even on rare occasions, surgery.[11] The prognosis in the pediatric and adolescent patient, in the absence of underlying structural abnormality, is quite good.

INDOMETHACIN-RESPONSIVE HEADACHES

The following four syndromes are infrequently seen in pediatric practice and may not be recognized by pediatricians. They are all specifically responsive to indomethacin. On close questioning, they are very different from migraine and from muscle contraction or tension headaches. They are usually unilateral and severe and respond to indomethacin.

Exertional Headaches

Exertional headaches are precipitated by exertion.[12] These headaches may be precipitated by coughing; sporting activities, such as running and swimming; and sexual activity. In the athlete, these headaches may interfere with training, practice, and performance. The headaches can occur during or after the activity and may be associated with nausea and vomiting, suggesting a life-threatening organic disorder. The headaches may be brief and generalized or sharply localized, and patients have described the pain as being similar to the blow of a hammer. The pain may last from 15 minutes to 12 hours. In the majority of instances, the headaches are benign. If patients, during the course of such a headache or shortly thereafter, have normal general physical examinations and neurologic examinations, an organic process is unlikely. Special attention should be paid to the patient's blood pressure.

The mechanism is thought to be due to increased intrathoracic pressure, sudden increase in blood pressure leading to extracranial dilation, and traction on the intracranial contents. High altitude, heat, humidity, and lack of training contribute to the headache.[13]

If the headaches occur only with exertion, imaging studies may not be necessary. This type of headache is to be differentiated from altitude headaches and effort migraine. If the patient has effort migraine, propranolol may be useful.

The treatment of these headaches should be conservative. In many patients, the effort headaches disappear spontaneously. Indomethacin can be used chronically and/or prior to specific activities. Improved conditioning can also decrease the frequency and severity of these headaches. Indeed, in one study, indomethacin completely controlled these headaches in 86% of patients.[14] If chronic indomethacin is to be used, monitoring for side effects is mandatory.

Cyclic Migraine

Cyclic migraine is a form of migraine that comes in cycles.[15] It has not been well reported in the pediatric and adolescent population. It has also been called cluster migraine, but it is not a form of cluster headache. The headache cycle averages 2 to 20 weeks with an average of 6 weeks. During the cycles, the headaches occur daily or several times per week. In between the migraine headaches, there may be a constant low-intensity headache. The majority of cycles last 6 weeks and are followed by headache-free intervals lasting many weeks to months. The majority of patients are female. The disorder may begin in the first or second decade, and more than 50% of the patients have a positive family history of migraine. In the absence of neurologic symptoms or signs, neuroimaging is seldom needed. The treatment of cyclic migraine has included lithium carbonate and indomethacin. The standard antimigraine therapy does not usually work. The pathogenesis of cyclic migraine is not known.

Chronic Paroxysmal Hemicrania

Chronic paroxysmal hemicrania (CPH) was described in 1974 by Sjaastad and Dale.[16] It is characterized by multiple daily attacks, usually five per day, which last anywhere from 5 to 30 minutes. They are unilateral and rarely alternate sides. The pain is described as severe, and autonomic phenomenon and other symptoms are usually lacking. The pain is most frequently localized to the eye or forehead above the eye. It may be precipitated by head movement. Chronic paroxysmal hemicrania has also been called atypical cluster headache. The disorder is usually seen in females and has only rarely been described in the pediatric literature.[17] The general physical and neurologic examinations between attacks are completely normal. During the attacks, the child is usually very uncomfortable and resists cooperating with the examiner. The pathogenesis of this disorder is unknown. This disorder responds dramatically to indomethacin, the beneficial effects appearing within 2 days. In many patients, if the indomethacin is discontinued the headaches reappear in several days.

Hemicrania Continua

Hemicrania continua was described in 1984 by Sjaastad and Spierings as another rare form of headache responsive to indomethacin.[18] This headache is characterized by a steady, nonparoxysmal, severe hemicrania localized to the frontal part of the head and not associated with nausea. Autonomic symptoms are not usually seen. There are no precipitating mechanisms, and the pathogenesis is not clear. The majority of patients affected are female and in the case reported by Zuckerman et al., the pain began during adolescence.[19] In these patients, there is no family history of headache.

Indomethacin, a potent anti-inflammatory and analgesic, was discovered in 1963.[20] There may be significant side effects associated with its chronic use. These include nausea, abdominal distress, and gastrointestinal bleeding. In addition, it may have central nervous system effects, including headache, dizziness, and mental confusion. Rarely, depression and psychosis have been reported. Hematologic side effects are uncommon. Renal side effects can be severe. The mechanism by which it improves the pain in the above-described headache syndrome is not known, but inhibition of prostaglandin synthesis has been implicated. In addition, it is well known that as an anti-inflammatory agent it decreases cerebral blood flow. Dosages as little as 25 mg per day may be helpful. The dosage should not exceed 150 mg per day. Patients chronically using indomethacin require careful monitoring.

ICE CREAM HEADACHE

Ice cream headache is the name applied to headache pain that is cold induced.[21] The International Headache Society (IHS) criteria defines it as a pain that develops during the ingestion of cold food or drink, lasts for less than 5 minutes, is felt in the middle of the forehead, is prevented by avoiding rapid swallowing of cold food and drink, and is not associated with organic disease. This type of headache occurs more frequently in patients who have migraine, but it can also occur in migraine-free patients. Raskin and Knittle found that 93% of migraine patients reported ice cream headaches, compared with 31% of nonheadache controls.[21] The majority of patients, in addition to headache, had toothache and pharyngeal pain. The headache was anterior and could either be unilateral or bilateral. It was of relatively short duration and in some patients quite severe. It is suggested that the pain is referred from the palate or teeth via the trigeminal nerve. The role of focal muscle contraction or vascular spasm is not known. The pain is self-limited, and only rarely is treatment indicated.

COUGH HEADACHE

Cough headache is considered by some a form of exertional headache and has also been described as "sneezing headache" and "laughing headache."[22] The IHS has defined benign cough headache as a bilateral headache of sudden onset that lasts less than 1 minute and is precipitated by coughing. It may be prevented by avoiding coughing. Because of reports associating this disorder with structural abnormalities, a neuroimaging study is suggested.[23] The etiology of this disorder is not clear. A transient increase in subarachnoid pressure and cerebrospinal fluid pressure has been postulated. It has been reported in children with chronic lung disease, such as cystic fibrosis.[24]

ICE PICK HEADACHE

Ice pick headache refers to brief, sharp, jabbing pains either as a single episode or in repeated episodes.[25] It has also been called "jabs and jolts headache." The IHS uses the following diagnostic criteria: pain exclusive to the distribution of the first division of the trigeminal nerve in the orbit, temple, and parietal area.[26] The pain is momentary, may occur several times daily, and is stabbing in nature. It occurs at irregular intervals and to make this diagnosis, a structural abnormality must be excluded. These headaches can be seen in patients free of other forms of headache or, more likely, in patients with migraine or cluster headaches. It is extremely uncommon in the pediatric and adolescent population. It has been treated successfully using indomethacin and in many cases disappears spontaneously.

ALTITUDE HEADACHE[13,27]

This headache is especially frequent in individuals who climb mountains and ski at high altitudes. It may be seen in acute mountain sickness along with the other primary symptoms of pulmonary edema and cerebral edema. The headache seen at high altitudes is usually associated with hypobaric hypoxia. The disorder usually occurs above 8,000 feet and increases in frequency as the elevation increases. The headache is usually described as generalized and throbbing and aggravated by exertion, coughing, and lying down. On examination, these patients may have retinal hemorrhages, papilledema, and confusion. The headache usually appears from 6 to 96 hours after arriving at high altitudes. The pathogenesis of this disorder has been explored by several authors.[28,29] Relief of the headache is obtained by descending to lower altitudes. Ergotamine may be effective, but oxygen inhalation is especially effective. The disorder may be prevented by acetazolamide, phenytoin, and dexamethasone.

FACIAL PAIN

Chronic facial pain is uncommon in children and adolescents. It is more likely seen in the aging population. Patients with sinusitis, dental disorders, cluster headaches, TMJ, CPH, and hemicrania continua may have facial headaches. Trigeminal neuralgia, temporal arteritis, and facial pain in patients with psychogenic disease are uncommon in the pediatric and adolescent population.[30] In the usual patient presenting with facial pain in an acute situation, it is usually related to sinusitis, dental disease, or trauma.

MELAS[31]

The combination of *m*itochondrial *e*ncephalomyopathy, *l*actic *a*cidosis, and *s*troke-like attacks, or MELAS, is rare. Patients may initially present with recurrent migraine-like headaches that are severe and prolonged and, at times, followed by seizures and stroke-like episodes. Episodic vomiting may occur. This disorder is maternally transmitted and due to a mitochondrial dysfunction. Many of the patients have short stature and by the time the diagnosis is made, have suffered from seizures, alternating hemiparesis, and focal neurologic abnormality. The syndrome begins between ages 3 and 11 years. Neuropathologic features in this disorder include ragged red fibers evident on muscle biopsy, lactic acidemia, and spongy degeneration of the brain. A defect in the respiratory chain in muscle mitochondria can be identified in most patients. In some patients, however, no biochemical defect has been identified. The clinical features, biochemistry, and molecular genetics of this disorder have recently been reviewed by Ciafaloni et al.[32] No treatment is available.

REFERENCES

1. Ekbom KA. Ergotamine tartrate orally in Horton's "histaminic cephalalgia" (also called Harris' "ciliary neuralgia"). Acta Psychiatr Scand 1947;46 (Suppl):106–113.

2. Kunkle EC, Pfeiffer JB Jr, Wilhoit WM, et al. Recurrent brief headache in "cluster" pattern. Trans Am Neurol Assoc 1952;77:240–243.

3. Kudrow L. Cluster Headache: Mechanism and Management. Oxford: Oxford University Press, 1980.

4. Ekbom K, Ahlborg B, Schéle R. Prevalence of migraine and cluster headache in Swedish men of 18. Headache 1978;18:9–19.

5. Maytal J, Lipton RB, Solomon S, Shinnar S. Childhood onset cluster headaches. Headache 1992;32:275–279.

6. Belfer ML, Kaban LB. Temporomandibular joint dysfunction. Pediatrics 1982;69:564–567.

7. Pillemer FG, Masek BJ, Kaban LB. Temporomandibular joint dysfunction and facial pain in children: an approach to diagnosis and treatment. Pediatrics 1987;80:565–570.

8. Hunter CR, Mayfield FH. Role of the upper cervical roots in the production of pain in the head. Am J Surg 1949;78:743–749.

9. Dugan MC, Locke S, Gallagher JR. Occipital neuralgia in adolescents and young adults. N Eng J Med 1962;267:1166–1172.

10. Rothner AD, Erenberg G, Cruse RP. Occipital neuralgia in adolescents (abstract). Ann Neurol 1988;24:330.

11. Poletti CE. Proposed operation for occipital neuralgia: C2 and C3 root decompression. Neurosurgery 1983;12:221–224.

12. Rooke DE. Benign exertional headaches. Med Clin North Am 1968;52:801–808.

13. Appenzeller O. Altitude headache. Headache 1972;12:126–129.

14. Diamond S. Prolonged benign exertional headache: its clinical characteristics and response to indomethacin. Headache 1982;22:96–98.

15. Medina JL, Diamond S. Cyclical migraine. Arch Neurol 1981;38:343–344.

16. Sjaastad O, Dale I. Evidence for a new(?), treatable headache entity. Headache 1974;14:105–108.

17. Broeske D, Lenn NJ, Cantos E. Chronic paroxysmal hemicrania in a young child: possible relation to ipsilateral occipital infarction. J Child Neurol 1993;8:235–236.

18. Sjaastad O, Spierings ELH. "Hemicrania continua": Another headache absolutely responsive to indomethacin. Cephalalgia 1984;4:65–70.

19. Zuckerman E, Hannuch SN, Carvalho D, et al. "Hemicrania continua": a case report. Cephalalgia 1987;7:171–173.

20. Hardman SG, Limbird LE, eds. Goodman and Gilman's The Pharmacological Basis of Therapeutics. 9th ed. St. Louis, MO: Pergamon Press, 1996, pp 633–635.

21. Raskin NH, Knittle SC. Ice cream headache and orthostatic symptoms in patients with migraine. Headache 1976;16:222–225.

22. Symonds C. Cough headache. Brain 1956;79:557–568.

23. Nightingle S, Williams B. Hindbrain hernia headache. Lancet 1987;1:731–734.

24. Katz RM. Cough syncope in children with asthma. J Pediatr 1970;77:48.

25. Raskin NH, Schwartz RK. Ice pick-like pain. Neurology 1980;30:203–205.

26. Classification and diagnostic criteria for headache disorders, cranial neuralgias and facial pain. Headache Classification Committee of the International Headache Society. Cephalalgia 1988;8(Suppl 7):39.

27. King AB, Robinson SM. Vascular headache of acute mountain sickness. Aerosp Med 1972;43:849–851.

28. Meehan RT, Zavala DC. The pathophysiology of acute high-altitude illness. Am J Med 1982;73:395–403.

29. Rootwelt K, Stokke KT, Nyberg-Hansen R, et al. Reduced cerebral blood flow in high altitude climbers. Scand J Clin Lab Invest 1986;46(Suppl 184): 107–112.

30. Raskin NH. Facial pain. In: Headache, 2nd ed. New York: Churchill Livingstone, 1988, pp 333–373.

31. Montagna P, Gallassi R, Medori R, et al. MELAS syndrome: characteristic migrainous and epileptic features and maternal transmission. Neurology 1988;38:751–754.

32. Ciafaloni E, Ricci E, Shanske S, et al. MELAS: clinical features, biochemistry, and molecular changes. Ann Neurol 1992;31:391–398.

Chapter 11

HEADACHE IN THE PEDIATRIC EMERGENCY DEPARTMENT

Donald W. Lewis

Headache is one of the more common presenting complaints to emergency departments (EDs). Each year, over 10 million patients visit their primary care physician or ED with a chief complaint of headache.[1] The overwhelming majority of headaches are benign in nature and can be accurately diagnosed on the basis of a careful history and physical examination. Headache can, however, be the initial symptom of life-threatening disorders, such as meningitis, intracranial hemorrhage, brain tumor, or hydrocephalus. It is, therefore essential for physicians to have a rational approach to the evaluation of a child or adolescent who presents to the ED with headache.

The purpose of this chapter is to review the etiologies, evaluation, and appropriate investigations for nontraumatic headache in the pediatric ED.

ETIOLOGIES

Three studies have examined the chief complaint of headache in the ED. Burton et al. reported that 1.3% of 53,988 visits to the Miami Children's Hospital ED during 1993 were for the evaluation of headache.[2] The records of 288 children, approximately half of the children, were retrospectively reviewed (Table 11–1).

Serious neurologic diseases were found in 6.6% and included 15 cases of viral meningitis, 1 shunt malfunction, 1 newly diagnosed hydrocephalus, and 1 patient with lymphoma metastatic to the brain. Crit-

Table 11–1   Spectrum of Diagnoses for Headache
at Miami Children's Hospital Emergency Department 1993

Diagnosis	Percentage
Viral illness	39.2
Sinusitis	16
Migraine	15.6
Post-traumatic disorder	6.6
Viral meningitis	5.2
Streptococcal pharyngitis	4.9
Tension	4.5
Other	7.7

Adapted from: Burton LJ, Quinn B, Pratt-Cheney JL, et al. Headache etiology in a pediatric emergency room. Pediatr Emerg Care 1997;13:1–4.

ically, all of these patients with serious neurologic conditions had abnormal findings on history or physical examination consistent with their diagnosis, except for a single patient with an unsuspected punctate hemorrhage following head trauma.

A second study, from Barcelona, investigated 140 patients who warranted admission to a short-stay unit with an incoming diagnosis of headache. Table 11–2 provides the most frequent diagnoses.

Central nervous system tumors were found in six patients, five of whom had papilledema. The authors conclude that complete neurologic examination must be performed, leaving further "complementary examinations for those cases where the patient history suggests organic alteration."[3]

The third study prospectively investigated the causes of acute headache in the pediatric ED and, similarly, found that viral infection with fever was the most common etiology. Table 11–3 shows the most frequent diagnoses in this population of 150 consecutive children who presented with the abrupt evolution of headache.[4]

Analysis of the clinical data revealed three important observations:

1.   Only 2 of 150 children had occipital headache; both had posterior fossa tumors. Occipital location of the pain must be considered strongly indicative of an organic pathology, specifically posterior fossa tumors.

Table 11–2   Most Frequent Diagnoses for Headache at a Short-Stay Unit

Diagnosis	Percentage
Infections	31
Tension	29
Migraine	21
Nonspecific	14
Other	5

Adapted from: Gutierrez de Pando L, Lopez Navarro JA, Fasheh Y, et al. Headache in a short-stay unit. A retrospective study. An Esp Pediatr 1999;50:562–565.

2. Over 60% of those children with surgically remediable conditions, brain tumors, or shunt malfunctions were unable to describe their pain. All other children in this study were easily able to do so. The lack of descriptive power must be viewed as a subtle sign of decreased verbal skill and disturbed mental status.

3. The neurologic examination is of great value. All patients with serious underlying pathologic processes had clear, objective neurologic signs including papilledema, ataxia, hemiparesis, and/or abnormal eye movements.

Table 11–3   Most Frequent Diagnoses for
Acute Headache in a Pediatric Emergency Department

Diagnosis	Percentage
Upper respiratory tract infection	57
Viral	(39)
Sinusitis	(9)
Streptococcal pharyngitis	(9)
Migraine without aura	18
Viral meningitis	9
Brain tumors (1 of each)	2.6
Medulloblastoma, pineal region germinoma	
Cerebellar astrocytoma, brain stem glioma	
Vertriculoperitoneal shunt malfunction	2
Intracranial hemorrhage (1 of each)	1.3
Hemorrhagic infarction	
Arteriovenous malformation	
Post-ictal headache	1.3
Postconcussive headache	1.3
Undetermined cause	7

The majority of headaches in children and adolescents presenting to the ED are due to common conditions such as upper respiratory infection (URI) and migraine. These diagnoses are confirmed by history and physical examination. In the three ED-based studies, all of the children with nontraumatic headache who had serious underlying conditions had demonstrable, objective findings on neurologic examination: alteration of consciousness, nuchal rigidity, papilledema, abnormal eye movements, ataxia, or hemiparesis. Therefore, abnormality on neurologic examination is the principle indication for neuroimaging. The value of a normal neurologic examination cannot be overstated.

CLINICAL APPROACH TO THE CHILD

The American College of Emergency Physicians issued a policy statement outlining the initial approach to adolescents presenting to the ED with a chief complaint of headache, excluding trauma-related headache.[5] This document emphasizes a logical sequence of history and physical examination and appropriate laboratory or imaging studies and must be viewed as the standard of care for ED physicians. Quality assurance assessment forms are included so that EDs can monitor their compliance. Health care providers are encouraged to review this publication.

Medical History

When evaluating a child with headache in the ED, the initial step is to gather history. The nature of the headache pain must be carefully addressed.

Table 11–4 shows the key information that should be obtained for a medical history.

Physical and Neurologic Examination

Following this history, a thorough physical and neurologic examination must be conducted and include those elements shown in Table 11–5.

Table 11–4   Key Information Required from Medical History

Temporal pattern or pace of onset of the headache (see Chapter 2)
    Acute, acute-recurrent, chronic progressive, chronic nonprogressive, or mixed

Duration

Frequency

Location

Quality and severity of pain

Exacerbating/alleviating factors

Response to treatments

Aura

Past history of headache

Changing quality/location/severity of pain

Family history of headache

Toxic exposure

Drugs (prescribed or recreational)
    Anticoagulants, anticonvulsants, birth control pills, asthma medicines, stimulants, antihypertensives, analgesics, carbon monoxide, lead

Trauma

Associated symptoms
    Fever
    Nausea, vomiting, photophobia, phonophobia

Neurologic symptoms
    Seizure, syncope, altered consciousness, declining school performance, neck pain or stiffness, vertigo, visual changes, diplopia, hearing loss or change, ataxia, disequilibrium, weakness, gait difficulty, back pain

Sinus or dental pain, nasal discharge, facial pain

Past medical history
    Neurosurgical procedures (ventriculoperitoneal shunt)
    Sinus disease
    Human immunodeficiency virus
    Endocrine disorders (hyperthyroidism)
    Congenital heart disease (increased risk for brain abscess or hypertension)
    Malignancy
    Coagulopathy
    Pregnancy and last menstrual period
    Rheumatologic or collagen vascular disease (lupus)
    Psychiatric disorders such as depression, suicide, anxiety disorder

Table 11–5   Required Elements of a Thorough Physical
and Neurologic Examination

Vital signs
   Blood pressure, pulse, respiration

General physical examination
   Nuchal rigidity, Kernig and/or Brudzinski's sign, sinus, throat, temporomandibular
   joint, dental, cervical lymph node tenderness, ocular pressure, visual acuity, pain with eye
   movement, proptosis

Funduscopic examination
   Papilledema, papillitis, retinal hemorrhage, venous pulsations

Cardiopulmonary examination

Skin rashes, petechiae, ecchymosis, needle tracts, neurocutaneous markers

Hepatosplenomegaly

Neurologic examination
   Mental status: speech, orientation, alertness, behaviour, changing level of consciousness
   Cranial nerves: pupillary reaction, eye movements, facial movement
   Motor: pronator drift, weakness, asymmetry
   Coordination: dysmetria, intention tremor, rapid alternating movement
   Deep tendon reflexes
   Gait: tandem gait (tightrope walking) and station, Romberg's sign

DIFFERENTIAL DIAGNOSIS

The most useful initial step in the development of a differential diagnosis is
to categorize the headache into one of the five temporal patterns (see Chapter 2). The patterns seen commonly in the ED—acute, acute recurrent, and
chronic progressive—will be discussed below. Chronic nonprogressive
(chronic daily headache) and the mixed pattern are the focus of Chapter 7.

Acute Headache

The most common cause of acute headache in children is URI with fever
(Figure 11–1). The presence of headache plus fever, however, must raise
concerns for meningitis, either bacterial or viral. If clinical examination
demonstrates nuchal rigidity without alteration of consciousness, signs of
increased intracranial pressure, or lateralizing features, lumbar puncture is
mandatory. If the mental status is altered or focal findings evident, then
cranial imaging is warranted prior to lumbar puncture, though blood cul-

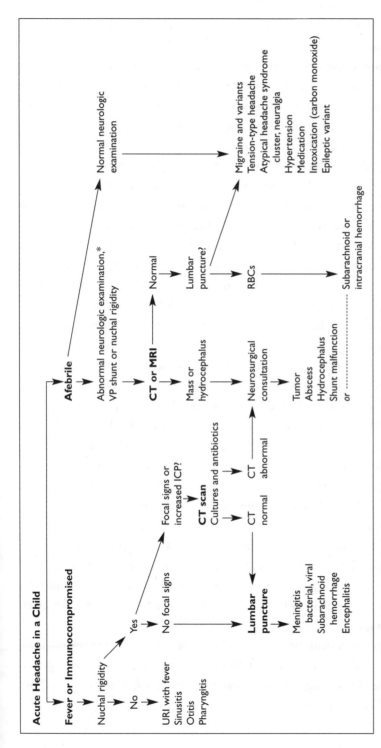

Figure 11-1 Evaluation of acute headache in a child. CT = computed tomography; MRI = magnetic resonance imaging; ICP = intracranial pressure; RBC = red blood cell; URI = upper respiratory infection; VP = ventriculoperitoneal. *5 key features: papilledema, abnormal eye movements, ataxia, hemiparesis, abnormal deep tendon reflexes. Adapted from: Dunn DW, Epstein LG. Acute headache. In: Dunn DW, Epstein LG, eds. Decision Making in Child Neurology. Toronto: B C Decker, 1987, p 70.

tures should be drawn and antibiotics empirically begun before the patient is transported for neuroimaging.

Another common, although overdiagnosed, cause for headache with fever is sinusitis and represents 9 to 16% of the causes of headache in the ED in children. If clinical history and physical examinations suggest acute sinusitis, sinus x-ray films or computed tomography scans (CT) of the sinuses are indicated.

Headache with or without fever in a patient with human immunodeficiency virus (HIV) infection or other immunocompromised state, requires an aggressive investigation for opportunistic central nervous system (CNS) infection, such as toxoplasmosis, cytomegalovirus (CMV), herpes simplex virus (HSV), fungi, atypical tuberculosis, or CNS lymphoma.

If history suggests a sudden, severe ("thunderclap") onset to the headache, subarachnoid hemorrhage (SAH) must be considered. Subarachnoid hemorrhage is rare in children and has three primary causes: (1) arteriovenous malformation (AVM) (cavernous angioma, venous angioma, capillary telangiectasia, and true AVM); (2) aneurysm (berry, giant, traumatic, and mycotic); and (3) miscellaneous causes including coagulopathy, sickle cell anemia, sympathomimetic intoxication, and leukemia.[6]

A noncontrasted head CT is warranted in those patients with suspected SAH. Small bleeds may be difficult to detect in which case lumbar puncture must be conducted. Comparison of the red cell count and supernatant between tubes 1 and 4 may be useful in the distinction of traumatic spinal tap from the hemorrhagic cerebrospinal fluid (CSF) of SAH. Coagulation studies and platelet counts must be checked.

A patient with a prior neurosurgical procedure, such as ventriculoperitoneal shunt placement, who develops headache must raise concerns for the possibility of shunt malfunction, with or without infection.

Should the history suggest potential exposure to carbon monoxide, the carboxyhemoglobin level needs to be evaluated and the patient given 100% oxygen.

The overwhelming majority of acute headaches in children and adolescents are due to common conditions such as URI with fever or migraine headache. These diagnoses are established by medical history and thorough physical and neurologic examination. In the three pediatric ED-based studies discussed earlier, all patients presenting with nontraumatic headache who were found to have serious underlying conditions had objective neurologic findings: alteration of consciousness, nuchal rigidity, papilledema, abnormal eye movements, ataxia, or hemiparesis. Therefore, abnormality on neurologic examination is the principle indication for neuroimaging. The value of a normal neurologic examination cannot be overstated (Table 11–6).

Acute Recurrent Headache

This pattern of headache implies episodes of headache separated by symptom-free intervals. The vast majority of acute recurrent headaches in children and adolescents are either migraine or tension-type headaches. Although there is some controversy as to which of these two is the most frequent, few would argue that the two represent the majority of episodic headache. Table 11–7 provides a differential diagnosis. Chapters 6 and 8 are dedicated to diagnosis and treatment options.

Table 11–6   Causes of Acute Headache

Paranasal infection
    Upper respiratory infection with fever
    Sinusitis
    Otitis
    Pharyngitis

Meningitis

Subarachnoid hemorrhage

Intracranial hemorrhage

Migraine

Hypertension

Trauma

Substance abuse
    Cocaine

Medications

Intoxications
    Carbon monoxide
    Lead

Table 11–7   Causes of Acute Recurrent Headache

Migraine
Migraine variants
Tension-type
Cluster
Neuralgias
Hypertension
Medications
Substance abuse
Epileptic variants

Chronic Progressive Headache

This temporal pattern describes headaches that gradually increase in frequency and severity over time. This is the most ominous of the five temporal profiles and carries with it the greatest likelihood of organic pathology (Table 11–8). When accompanied by symptoms and signs of increased intracranial pressure, an aggressive evaluation for space occupying lesions must be conducted.

Several associated historic clues may further heighten the chances of tumor, abscess, hematoma, or vascular anomaly. Morning headache or headaches that awaken the child from sleep are classic symptoms of the dependent edema of intracranial lesions and obstructive hydrocephalus. Likewise, nocturnal or morning emesis, with or without headache, suggest increased intracranial pressure and are particularly common symptoms of tumors arising near the floor of the fourth ventricle. Between headaches, behavioral or mood changes, some of which may be subtle, are described by parents. Cognitive changes—demonstrated by declining school performance—can, on occasion, be the presenting complaint. Careful history can ferret out these associated features.

There is no invariable brain tumor headache profile. It is essential to recognize this temporal pattern of escalating headache frequency and severity that then dictates a course of action, usually, neuroimaging with magnetic resonance imaging (MRI). The MRI is much more useful than CT in this setting since it permits better visualization and definition of posterior fossa anatomy.

In 1991, the findings of The Childhood Brain Tumor Consortium study were reported. Detailed analysis of over 3,000 children with brain tumors demonstrated that 98% had at least 1 of 5 signs including papilledema, ataxia, hemiparesis, abnormal eye movements, or depressed reflexes.[7] Fifty percent of the patients had 5 signs at diagnosis. Five key points on neurologic examination must be documented when assessing a child with chronic progressive headache: (1) optic discs, (2) eye movements, (3) pronator drift, (4) tandem gait, and (5) deep tendon reflexes (DTRs).

Papilledema may be difficult to appreciate in the young or uncooperative child. Even in experienced hands, direct ophthalmoscopy can be a challenge. In this historic setting, the challenge must be overcome either by

Table 11–8   Chronic Progressive Headache

Hydrocephalus
    Obstructive
    Communicating
Neoplasm
    Medulloblastoma
    Cerebellar astrocytoma
    Ependymoma
    Pineal region tumor
    Craniopharyngioma
    Astrocytoma
Brain abscess
Subdural hematoma
Chronic meningitis
    Cryptococcal
    Lyme disease
Pseudotumor cerebri
Aneurysm
Malformations
    Chiari
    Dandy-Walker
Hypertension
Medications
    Birth control pills
    Stimulants
Intoxications
    Carbon monoxide
    Lead poisoning

Table 11–9   Chronic Progressive Headache Summary: Key Points

No invariable brain tumor headache profile

Chronic progressive headache strongly suggestive of organic pathology

Key symptoms
    Nocturnal or morning headache
    Nocturnal or morning vomiting
    Aggravation by Valsalva's maneuver or exertion
    Seizures

Key signs
    Papilledema
    Cranial nerve palsies
    Ataxia
    Focal signs, motor or sensory

Look for neurocutaneous syndromes

If the discs need to be seen, do so

Always check the head circumference

performance of a dilated examination or by obtaining ophthalmologic consultation. Table 11–9 provides a summary of the key points regarding chronic progressive headache.

When to Image in the Evaluation of Headache

Table 11–10 outlines when imaging is necessary for evaluating headache in children.

Table 11–10   Imaging for the Evaluation of Headache

High priority
    Chronic progressive pattern
    Acute headache
        Worst headache of life
        Thunderclap headache
    Abnormal neurologic examination
    Focal neurologic symptoms
    Presence of ventriculoperitoneal shunt
    Presence of neurocutaneous syndrome (neurofibromatosis or tuberous sclerosis)
    Age < 3 years

Moderate priority
    Headaches or vomiting on awakening
    Unvarying location of headache
    Meningeal signs

CONCLUSION

The majority of headaches during childhood and adolescence presenting to the ED are caused by self-limited illnesses or medically remediable conditions. Serious disorders, such as tumors, meningitis, hemorrhages, or abscesses, are infrequent and, when present, are accompanied by objective neurologic signs.

The most important neurodiagnostic tool in the evaluation of headache in children is a careful history. Exploration of the onset, pace, and evolution of the symptom complex will dictate the scope and urgency of ancillary testing.

CASE PRESENTATIONS

Case 1

A 15-year-old wrestler was competing in the regional final for his weight division and in the dominant position over his less-skilled opponent "riding" when he experienced a sudden stabbing pain in his right posterior temple. He felt momentarily stunned and his competitor quickly took advantage and pinned him, winning the match. The victor and spectators were celebrating, not noticing the loser was lying on the mat holding his head, writhing in pain. The coach went over to console the young man and recognized that he was confused and not using his left arm. Emergency medical services transported him to the ED. His physical examination revealed the following:

Blood pressure 145/92, pulse 150, temperature 37.7
Awake; knew his name, age, location, and outcome of match
No nuchal rigidity
Left visual field inattention
Right gaze preference
Optic discs normal with preserved venous pulsations
Depression of left nasolabial fold
Left pronator drift
Exaggerated DTRs on the left
Left extensor plantar response

This young man experienced an acute stabbing pain on the right side of his head with accompanying signs localizing to the right temporal parietal region.

The differential diagnosis must include: intracranial hemorrhage; vascular malformations such as cavernous angioma, venous angioma, arteriovenous malformation, capillary telangiectasis; aneurysm such as congenital "berry" aneurysms (associated with aortic coarctation and polycystic kidney); arterial dissection; coagulopathy; sympathomimetic intoxication from cocaine and amphetamine; subdural hemorrhage; hypertension; hypertensive hemorrhage; and exertional migraine.

An emergent noncontrasted head CT scan disclosed a 2.5-cm intraparenchymal parietal hematoma with a second left frontal 0.75-cm calcified lesion. The MRI confirmed multiple cavernous angiomas.

The wrestler was diagnosed with an intracranial hemorrhage secondary to occult cavernous angioma. This is often a familial, autosomal dominant condition.

Case 2

A mother was preparing dinner when she realized there were some ingredients she was missing. She hastily bustled the 5-year-old twin girls into her teenage son's reconditioned noisy VW bus and rushed to the market. The twins didn't want to go in, so she left them in the car with the heater and engine running since it was a cold day. She ran into her minister while shopping and chatted for about 5 to 10 minutes. After completing her shopping, she returned to the vehicle and the twins were asleep. After she returned home she had difficulty arousing the girls and left them in the car to get dinner in the oven. On returning she was able to wake the girls up but they were nauseated and complained of severe global headache. Mother rushed them to the ED thinking they may have "gotten into something" in her son's car. Continuing that line of thought, the ED gave them ipecac followed by charcoal. Urine toxic screens were negative. The ED personnel then performed CT scans on both girls which were normal. The girls' examination revealed the following:

Blood pressure 100/70, pulse 120, oxygen saturation 100% on room air

Mental status: prefer to sleep, arouse to voice fully oriented
Cranial nerves: normal
Motor, sensory, appendicular coordination, and DTRs normal
Refused to stand up or walk

These previously healthy twins simultaneously developed headache and nausea. The ED team appropriately considered a common intoxication with sympathomimetic agents, such as cocaine or amphetamines; however an environmental exposure was most likely. Given that the VW bus was old and noisy, it probably had a poor exhaust system. The ED determined that the girls were exposed to carbon monoxide (CO).

Children are particularly vulnerable to the effects of CO. One of the earliest symptoms is headache. Exposure from kerosene space heaters, faulty ventilation systems, or automobile or boat fumes can have fatal consequences. The diagnosis can be quickly established by measurement of the carboxyhemoglobin level.

Case 3

A 7-year-old girl presented to the ED with periodic headaches. Once a week, usually in the morning before breakfast or late in the evening before bed, she would tell her mother the she suddenly saw balloons off to her right. The images were brightly colored and gradually faded away, after which she would complain of an intense parieto-occipital headache with nausea and an intense desire to rest.

Her medical history was otherwise quite benign. Her grandmother had migraine and one cousin had epilepsy. Her examination was normal.

She was diagnosed as having migraine with aura and begun on cyproheptadine. This was unsuccessful, as was propranolol.

Migraine with aura represents less than 20% of migraine in children. Those children who do experience an aura, do so inconsistently—not every migraine is accompanied by aura. The typical aura is a binocular scotoma and, infrequently, hallucination. The aura appears gradually, not abruptly as with the girl.

Young children typically have their migraine attacks late in the afternoon. Older adolescents will suffer their events at earlier hours of the day, as with adults.

The abruptness of onset of this unusual well-formed aura occurring at an odd time of day must raise suspicions of alternate diagnoses.

An electroencephalogram disclosed sleep enhanced, left occipital spikes, consistent with benign occipital epilepsy. She was begun on carbamazepine at 20 mg per kg, with prompt cessation of events.

Case 4

A 14-year-old boy hated his piano lessons. Every parental attempt to motivate him was unsuccessful. Eventually, grandmother contracted a $10 bribe to gain his cooperation.

Each Thursday, after school he would reluctantly head off to his lesson and return an hour later quite excited and talkative. About 20 to 30 minutes later he would complain of a severe headache, occasionally vomit, and become very agitated. Initially, all assumed this to be avoidance behavior and ignored it for about 2 months.

After a particularly bad headache, medical attention was sought and he was noted to have a blood pressure of 145/100 and pulse of 150 beats per minute, during a headache. Hypertensive work-up, including urinary catachols, was unrevealing. Neurologic examination was normal.

The piano teacher unexpectantly became ill and had to suspend lessons for a month. During the month, our patient had no headaches, further convincing his family the attacks were avoidance.

For his birthday, his loving grandmother gave him $50. He presented to the ED following a 20-minute generalized convulsion. The CT scan was normal, but the urinary toxic screen was positive for cocaine.

He later admitted that after each piano lesson he would spend his $10 bribe on crack cocaine.

Case 5

An active 5-year-old presented to the ED with 6 weeks of intermittent frontal headaches. For the prior 3 weeks he had been complaining of daily headache, but his mother attributed this to his grandmother's recent death. Through the past week, the child had begun to crawl upstairs. Even with his hand held, he would not walk up steps. He continued to run down steps with great agility and all his other activities seemed normal. His examination revealed the following:

Head circumference > 98%
General examination is normal
Mental status is normal
Cranial nerves: normal optic discs
Eye movements: limitation of vertical gaze
Motor, sensory, coordination, gait, and DTRs normal

The center for vertical gaze is located in the rostral midbrain. The aqueduct of Sylvius courses through this region, so compressive processes would not only inhibit upward gaze but produce obstructive hydrocephalus. Pineal region tumors, such as a germinoma, pineoblastoma, and astrocytoma, would be the leading considerations.

Aqueductal stenosis (AS) must also be considered. The classic "sunset" sign of AS is produced by pressure at the region of stenosis in the periaqueductal zone.

A noncontrasted CT scan disclosed dilated lateral and third ventricles with a normal-size fourth ventricle. No masses were identified. The MRI confirmed aqueductal narrowing and did not demonstrate midbrain tumor.

Aqueductal stenosis commonly presents in infancy with macrocephaly, full fontanelle, and restriction of vertical gaze with lid retraction (sunset sign) but may cause obstructive hydrocephalus at any age. Midbrain pilocytic astrocytomas, an unusually indolent brain stem tumor, may be difficult to detect on CT scan alone; therefore MRI is advisable, particularly when hydrocephalus due to suspected AS occurs at unusual ages.

Case 6

An appearance-conscious 14-year-old girl began to complain of bitemporal pounding headache each morning. Her parents were convinced she was attempting to avoid school since her acne had blossomed. The headaches were quite intense in the morning but remitted by noon. By the afternoon hours she was able to engage in her usual activity of talking on the phone.

The CT scan was normal. Psychologic consultation was sought and "school phobia" diagnosed. She was placed on a "home bound" school program since she had missed more than 3 weeks of classes. Later, she noticed episodes of "fuzzy" vision lasting just minutes but which were not strictly time-linked to her headaches. Her examination revealed the following:

Weight 75%, Height 25%
Neurologic examination normal except bilateral papilledema
Lumbar puncture opening pressure > 400 mm H_2O
Lymphocyte 1
Protein 14 mg/dL
Glucose 47 mg/dL

The patient was diagnosed with pseudotumor cerebri (PTC).

PTC is common in adolescents and, although often idiopathic, may be precipitated by a variety of processes including endocrinopathies, infection, collagen vascular diseases, and drugs.

This young lady had been placed on a tetracycline derivative about 2 weeks before developing her headaches. Additionally, she had read in her teen magazines that vitamin A helped acne. She doubled up her antibiotic and took a minimum of four 25K-units vitamin A tablets per day.

Cessation of both the antibiotic and the vitamin A supplements coupled with 4 weeks of acetazolamide resulted in prompt resolution of her disc edema and headaches.

Case 7

A 9-year-old boy presented with 3 months of gradually increasing headache and vomiting, usually in the morning. For the past week his headaches had awoken him from sleep. He had been evaluated weekly by his family practice physician who serially recorded "Neuro: WNL, Non-lateralizing" examination.

After 4 weeks, his parents sought another opinion from a pediatrician who similarly found "no focal findings," diagnosed sinusitis, and prescribed Augmentin for 3 weeks.

After 2 weeks without improvement, the mother took her son to an optometrist who recognized disc changes. He was referred to the ED where "papilledema" and "trouble with tandem gait" were found.

An MRI scan disclosed a large midline posterior fossa mass. The differential diagnosis included medulloblastoma, ependymoma, and cerebellar astrocytoma.

The majority of brain tumors in childhood are midline processes (e.g., medulloblastoma, cerebellar astrocytoma, ependymoma, pineal region tumors, craniopharyngioma). Therefore, there may be little in the way of "lateralizing" physical findings (the myth of the "nonfocal examination"). It is essential, then, to recognize that this chronic progressive pattern, particularly when coupled with the nocturnal or early morning predominance, is a cardinal symptom of increased intracranial pressure.

REFERENCES

1. Rassmussen BK, Jensen R, Schroll M, et al. Epidemiology of headache in a general population—a prevalance study. J Clin Epidemiol 1991;44: 1147–1157.
2. Burton LJ, Quinn B, Pratt-Cheney JL, et al. Headache etiology in a pediatric emergency room. Pediatr Emerg Care 1997;13:1–4.
3. Gutierrez de Pando L, Lopez Navarro JA, Fasheh Y, et al. Headache in a short stay unit. A retrospective study. An Esp Pediatr 1999;50:562–565.
4. Lewis DW, Qureshi FA. Acute headache in the pediatric emergency department. Headache 2000;40:200–203.
5. American College of Emergency Physicians. Clinical policy for the initial approach to adolescents and adults presenting to the emergency department with a chief complaint of headache. Ann Emerg Med 1996;27:821–844.
6. Getzoff M, Goldstein B. Spontaneous subarachnoid hemorrhage in children. Pediatr Rev 1999;4;141.
7. The epidemiology of headache among children with brain tumors. Headache in children with brain tumors. The Childhood Brain Tumor Consortium. J Neurooncol 1991;10:31–46.

INDEX

Abdominal migraine, 79
Acetaminophen, 96
    dosage, acute, *88*
Activities, 131–132
Acute headache, *174*
    causes, *171*
    evaluation, *169*
    recurrent, 171, *172*
Acute post-traumatic headache, 40
Acute therapy as preventive therapy, 100
Adduction defect, 73
Agitation, 76
Alcohol as trigger, 154
"Alice in Wonderland" syndrome, 65, 67,
    75–76
    abrupt appearance of, 66
Allergy, 24, 25
Alternating hemiplegia, *67*, 69–71
Altitude headache, 159–160
Amerge, 92
American Migraine Study prevalence, 12
Amitriptyline, 78, 148
    dosage, preventive, *104,* 105–106
Amnesia, 76, 144
Analgesics, 96–98, 148
    avoiding overuse, 128–129
    dosage, acute, *88*
    rebound headaches with, 96
Aneurysm, 41, 42, 74
Anterior visual pathway migraine, 74
Anticonvulsants as preventive therapy,
    104–105
Antidepressants as preventive therapy,
    105–106
Antiemetics, 93–96, 148
Antihistamines as preventive therapy, 107
Aphasia, 76
Aqueductal stenosis, 180
Arnold-Chiari malformation, 36–37
Ataxia, 24, 36, 40, 65, 71, *72,* 77
    abrupt appearance of, 66
Attention deficit disorder (ADD)
    with stimulants for, *22, 23*
Aura, 3, 61, 65, *67*
    headache without, 63, *67*
    incidence, 8
    stroke-like, 68
Autoimmune disorders, 41
Axocet, *88*

Balance difficulty, *23,* 77
Basilar artery migraine, 71
Basilar impression, 72
Behavior, 7, 20, *23,* 41
    change in, 63
Behavior disorders, 143, 144
Behavioral therapies, 133–136
Behavioral treatment, 123
Benign intracranial hypertension, 43
Benign paroxysmal torticollis, 77–78
Benign paroxysmal vertigo, *67,* 77
    variant, 78
β-Blockers, 148
    as preventive therapy, 107–108
Bias
    recall, 2
    referral, 2
    selection, 2
Bickerstaff migraine, 71
Biofeedback, 135–136
    thermal, 135
Birth control pills, *22*
Blackouts, 75
Blindness, 64, 76
Blood dyscrasia, 42
Blood pressure, 26, 156
Brain abscess, 27
    emergency evaluation, 39
Brain tumor, 41, 66, 163, 180–181
Brudzinski's sign, 38

Café-au-lait spots, 26
Calcitonin gene-related peptide (CGRP),
    48–50
Calcium channel blockers,
    as preventive therapy, 109
    side effects, 109
Cardiac arrhythmia, 108
Case presentations, 96–98
    activities, 131–132
    analgesic overuse, 128–129
    chronic daily, 118–119
    emergency 1: sports injury, 175–176
    emergency 2: fumes, 176–177
    emergency 3: epilepsy, 177–178
    emergency 4: substance, 178
    emergency 5: aqueductal stenosis, 180
    emergency 6: pseudotumor cerebri, 180
    emergency 7: brain tumor, 180–181

school issues, 137–138
sleep patterns, 129–130
Cat-scratch disease, 39
Caudal cells, 51
Causative circumstances, *22*
Central nervous system (CNS)
  disturbance, 148
  infection, 66
  tumor, 164–165
Cerebral blood flow, 53
Cerebral edema, 145
Childhood periodic syndromes, 77–79
Chronic daily headache, 116–125, 143
  case presentation, 118–119
  classification, 116–119
  comorbid, 118
  diagnostic workup, 121–122
  duration, 117
  etiologic factors, 121
  management, *123*
  mixed, 119
  patient examination, 120
  patient history, 120
  physiology, 121
  prevalence, 116
  prognosis, 123
  stress in, 121
  tension-type, 117
  treatment, 121–123
Chronic paroxysmal hemicrania, 157
Chronic progressive, 172–174
Classification, Silberstein's, *111*
Clonidine as preventive therapy,110
Clumsiness, 71
Cluster headache, *21–22*, 81–82, 143, 146,
    153–154
  characterization, 153
  pain in, *22*
  pathophysiology, 52
Codeine, 96
Cognitive therapy, 133–134
Coma scale, *142*
Comorbid headache, 118
Computed tomography (CT), 28–29, 146, 172
Concentration difficulty, 143
Confusion, 65, *68*, *72*, 160
  abrupt appearance of, 66
  acute 76
Confusional migraine, 76–77
Congenital malformations, emergency
    evaluation, 36–37
Conjunctival injection, *82*
Consciousness
  altered, 28, 42

loss of, 28, 42
Cortex, 52
Cough headache, 156, 159
Cranial bruit, 26
Cranial nerve examination, 26
Cravings, 63
Cyclic migraine, 157
Cyclic vomiting syndrome, 77, 78–79
  variant of, 79
Cyproheptadine, 78, 148
  dosage, preventive, 107
  as preventive therapy, *104*, 107

Database, *21–23*
Dehydration, 42
Dementia, 69
Depacon, 104
Depakote, dosage, preventive, *104*, 105
Depakote ER, 104
Depression, 9, 63, 143, 144
  symptoms of, 26
D.H.E., 45, 93, 148
Diabetes, 25, 108
Diagnostic workup, 121–122
  indications for, 121
Diary, 20
Diet, 132
  as preventive therapy, 101
Differential diagnosis, 28
Dihydroergotamine, 93–96, 148
  administration, 93, *94*
  with antiemetic, 94
  with metoclopramide, *94*, 95
  patient history, 94
  protocols, *93*
  side effects, *95*
  titration, 95
Diphenhydramine, dosage, 95
Diplopia, 37, 71, 73
  sudden, 72
Disorientation, 76
Divalproex sodium as preventive therapy,
    103, 104–105
Dizziness, 71, 143, 144, 155
Dotarizine
  dosage, preventive, *104*
  as preventive therapy, 103
Drug-induced
  illicit, *23*, 39–40
  medications, *23*, 39–40
Duration of attacks, *3*, 5, 22
Dysarthria, *72*

Ear infections, 25

Elavil
  dosage, preventive, *104*, 148
Electroencephalogram (EEG), 28, 65
Eletriptan, 92, 98
Emboli, 41
Emergency evaluation, 27, 66
  acute headache, 168–171
  aqueductal stenosis, 180
  brain abscess, 39
  brain tumor, 180–181
  case presentations, 175–181
  chronic progressive headache, 172–174
  clinical approach, 166–168
  congenital malformations, 36–37
  differential diagnosis, 168–174
  encephalitis, 38
  epilepsy, 177–178
  etiologies, 163–166
  evaluation, *169*
  fumes, 176–177
  imaging, *175*
  infection, 37
  medical history, 166, *167*
  meningitis, 38
  most frequent diagnoses, *165*
  neoplasms, 40–41
  neurologic examination, 166–168
  physical examination, 166–168
  pseudotumor cerebri, 43, 180
  secondary headaches, 36–43
  sinusitis, 38
  sports injury, 175–176
  substance abuse, 178
  substance-induced, 39–40
  trauma, 40
  vascular disorders, 41–43
Emotional factors, 25
Encephalitis, emergency evaluation, 38
Epilepsy, 24, 69, 177–178
Ergot alkaloids, 92–96
Ergotamine compounds, 110
Ergotamines, 80, 154, 160
Esgic*plus*, 88
Evaluation, 20–32
  emergency, 27–28, 163–181
  history, 20–25
  laboratory, 28
  neuroimaging, 28–30, *175*
  neurologic, 26–27
  physical, 26
Excitement, 78
Exercise, 132–133
  as preventive therapy, 101
Exertional headaches, 156
Eye infections, 25
Eye movements, abnormal, 26

Eyelid edema, *82*

Facial pain, 154, 160
Familial hemiplegic migraine, 68–69
Family history, 3, 6, *23*, 24, 61, 76, 78
Family therapy, 138–139
Feeding problems, 9
Fever, 26
  aspirin during, 80
  with stiff neck, 27, 38
  with tachycardia, 37
Fioricet, *88*
Fluid on scalp, 26
Flunarizine, 108–109
Fluoxetine, dosage, preventive, 106
Focal deficits, *70*
Focal neurologic symptoms, 38, 39, 42, 69, *70*
Follow-up, 29–30
Fontanel, bulging, 38
Forgetfulness, *23*
Frequency, 14, 22
  changing, *22*
  increasing, 14
Fumes, 176–177

Gabapentin as preventive therapy, 103
Gait abnormalities, 26, 37
Glasgow coma scale, *142*, 146
Grayouts, 75

Head examination, 26
Head injury, 142–152
Head tilt, 77–78
Head trauma, 25, 76
  acute post-traumatic headache, 40
  penetrating, 39
Headache calendars, 99–100
Headache disability, 102
Headache medications causing headache, 39–40
Hearing loss, *72*
Heart murmurs, 25
Hematomas, 42
Hematuria, 42
Hemicrania continua, 117
  description, 158
Hemiparesis, 65, 68, 69, 76
  abrupt appearance of, 66
Hemiplegic migraine
  signs and symptoms, *68*
Hemisyndrome migraine
  signs and symptoms, *68*
Hemorrhage, 27, 41
  CT for, 28
  intracranial, 66, 176
Herpes encephalitis, 39

Histamine, 154
History, 20–25, 119–120
Hydrocephalus, 27, 66, 36, 163
  shunt malfunction, 37
5-Hydroxytryptamine agonists, 89
Hypertension, 23, 24, 27, 41–42, 145
Hyperventilation, 26
Hypnosis, 134–135
  self, 107, 135

Ibuprofen, dosage, acute, 88
Ice cream headache, 158–159
  IHS criteria, 158
Ice pick headache, 159
Imitrex, dosage, acute, 91
  efficacy of, 89
Incidence, definition, 7
Inderal, dosage, preventive, 105, 107
Indomethacin
  chronic use, 156, 158
  dosage, 158
  side effects, 158
Indomethacin-responsive headaches, 155–160
Infection, emergency evaluation, 37
Initiating factors, 21
Intermittence, 21
International Headache Society (IHS)
  criteria
    classification, 67
    revised, 3, 4, 62
    sensitivity, 4–6
  cough headache, 159
  ice cream headache, 158
  ice pick headache, 159
  migraine, 1–7, 3, 15, 60–62
  post-traumatic, 144
  prevalence, 9–15
  secondary headaches, 34
Intoxication, 66
Intracranial hemorrhage, 163
Intracranial pressure, increased, 21, 27, 36, 41, 43
  symptoms of, 23, 24
Irritability, 37, 38, 63

Juvenile migraine, 76

Kernig's sign, 38

Laboratory tests, 28
Lacrimation, 82, 153
Lactic acidosis, 69
Lesion, space-occupying
  imaging for, 29
Lethargy, 23, 36–38, 41, 63
Lifestyle modifications, 129–133

Lyme disease, 39

Macrocephaly, 36–37
Magnetic resonance arteriography, 29
Magnetic resonance imaging (MRI), 28–29, 146, 154, 172
Magnetic resonance venography, 29
Massage, 143
Maxalt, dosage, acute, 91, 92
Medical history, 24–25
  emergency, 167
Medication
  action of, 49, 51
  follow-up, 29–30
  future prospects, 50
  understanding, 29
Medication overuse, 14–15
MELAS, 69, 70, 160–161
  neuropathologic features, 160
Memory disorder, 143
Menarche
  prevalence of migraine during, 12
Meningismus, 42
Meningitis, 27, 29, 164
  emergency evaluation, 38
Mental status changes, 38
Meperidine hydrochloride, 97
Metoclopramide, 96
  diphenhydramine with, 95
  dosages, 94
  side effects, 95
Migraine equivalents, 77
Migraine
  abdominal, 79
  with aura, 65, 67, 75
  without aura, 63–64, 67, 97
  basilar, 67, 71–73, 76–78
    signs and symptoms, 72
    SPECT during, 72
  characterization, 60
  classifications, 1–19, 67
  confusional, 76–77
  cyclic pattern, 64
  definitions, 1–6, 15, 61
  diagnostic criteria, 3–7
  duration, 63
  epidemiology, 1–19
  familial hemiplegic, 67, 68–69
  features of, 2, 3
    inability to report, 4
  frequency, 14, 63
  genetics of, 68–69
  hemisyndrome, 68
  IHS criteria, 1–7, 61, 67
  IHS revised criteria, 3, 62
  incidence, 7–9

juvenile, 76
morning occurrence, 64
ophthalmoplegic, *67*, 73–74
    urgency, 74
pathophysiology, 47–59
prevalence, 9–15
    increasing, 13
prodromal features, 63
retinal, *67*, 74–75
studies of, 1–19
symptoms, *64*
transformed, 14–15
trauma-triggered, 76
understanding, 47
variants, 65–80, 76
    management of, 80
    pathogenesis, 66
Miosis, *82*, 153
Mood changes, 63
Mountain sickness, 159
Movements, abnormal, 28, 69–70
Multiple daily headaches, 157
Muscle contraction headache, *22*, 81
    pain in, *22*

Naproxen sodium
    dosage, acute, *88*
    dosage, preventive, 110
Naratriptan, 92
Nasal congestion, *82*
Nasal symptoms, 153
National Health Interview Study (NHIS)
    prevalence, 12
Nausea, 3, *21*, *23*, 36, 60–62, *72*, 79, 155, 156
    with photophobia, 97
Neck
    pain, 38, 51
    stiffness, 27, 38
Neoplasms
    emergency evaluation, 40–41
    incidence, 40–41
Neuroanatomic process, *48*
Neurocutaneous disorder, 121
Neuroimaging, 28–30, *175*
Neurologic examination, 26–27
Neuropeptide studies, 50
Neuropsychologic testing
    postconcussion syndrome, 146–147
New persistent daily headache, 117
Nimodipine, 109
Nonpharmocologic measures, *103*
    as preventive therapy, 101–102
Nonprogressive
    chronic, *23*
    daily, *21*

Nonsteroidal anti-inflammatory drugs
    (NSAIDs), *23*
    long-term use, 110
    for post-traumatic headache, 147–148
    as preventive therapy, 109–110
Nortriptyline, dosage, preventive, *104*, 106, 148
Nuchal rigidity, 38
Number of attacks, *3*
Nystagmus, 69, 77

Occipital headache, 22, 164
    causes of, 22
Occipital neuralgia, 155
Occult cavernous angioma, 176
Ocular migraine, 74
Office setting, 34–36
Onset, 21
Ophthalmic migraine, 74
Ophthalmoparesis, 65–66, 73–74
    abrupt appearance of, 66
Ophthalmoplegic migraine, *67*, 73–74
Opioids, 97
Optic atrophy, 26
Organic headaches. *See* Secondary headaches
Organomegaly, 26
Oxygen, 154, 160

Pain, *3*, 63
    abdominal, 25, 63, 79
    band-like, *22*
    bifrontal, *22*, 62, 97
    bilateral, 51, 62, 81, 117, 118
    bitemporal, *22*, 62
    chronic, 20
    intensity, 6
    limb, 25
    location, *22*
    neck, 51
    non-pulsating, *81*
    occipital, 62
    pressing, 117
    pulsatile, 6
    quality, *22*
    reactions to, 20
    skull, 154
    throbbing, 6, 60
    thunderclap, 170
    tightening, 117
    unilateral, 5–6, *22*, 61, 117, 153, 154, 157
    vertex, *22*
Pain sites, 50
Pain systems, 52
Pallor, 64, 71
Pamelor, dosage, preventive, *104*, 148
Papilledema, 37, 42, 164

Paralysis, 69–70
Parental distress, 139
Paresthesias, 76
Paroxysmal hemicrania, *22*
   chronic, 157
   pain in, 22
Patient education sheets, *130*
Patient interview, 20
Periactin, dosage, preventive, *104*
Personality change, *23*, 41
Personality tests, 29
Phonophobia, *3*, 6, 60–63, 81, 100, 118
Photophobia, *3*, 6, 60–63, 81, 100, 118
   with nausea, 97
Photopsia, 75
Physical examination, 26, 120
Pizotifen, 110
Plasma protein extravasation, 49
Platybasia, 72
Post-traumatic headache, 142–152
   age and injury, 148
   brainstem, 146
   coma scale, 142–143, 146
   diagnosis, 144–145
   diagnostic evaluations, 146
   IHS guideline, 144
   neuropsychologic testing, 146–147
   prognosis, 149
   symptoms of, *145*
   treatment, 147–149
Postconcussion syndrome, 142–152
Predictors, 9
Pressing tightness, 81
Prevalence, 9–15
   American Migraine Study, 12
   increasing, 13
Preventive goals, 87
Preventive therapy strategies, 98–111
   medications, 101–111
   treatment period, 110–111
Primary headache disorders, 1
Prochlorperazine maleate, 96
Promethazine hydrochloride, 96
Propranolol
   contraindication, 108
   dosage, preventive, *104*, 107–108
   hypertension dosage, 107
   possible side effects, 108
Pseudotumor cerebri, 145, 180
   aura in, 64
   blindness, 64
   emergency evaluation, 43, 180
   imaging for, 29
Psychiatric comorbidity, risk of, 138
Ptosis, 73, *82*, 153

Pulmonary problems, 25

Rash, 26
Rebound headache, 15
Recurrence, 116
   acute, 171
Relaxation therapies, 134–135, 136
Remission rate, 14
Respiratory irregularity, 70
Retinal hemorrhage, 42, 160
Retinal migraine, *67*, 74–75
Retinal pallor, 75
Rhinorrhea, *82*, 153
Rickettsial disease, 39
Rizatriptan
   dosage, acute, *91*, 92
   efficacy, 92, 98
   side effects, 92

Salicylates, Reye's syndrome and, 88
Scalp tenderness, 26, 155
School issues, 25, 143
   addressing, 136–138
   assessing, 29
   homebound program caution, 138
Scotoma, 65, 75
Secondary headaches, 33–46
   IHS categories, 33, *34*
   office setting, 34–36
Second impact syndrome, 145
Seizures, 38, 41, 160
Self-hypnosis, 107, 135
Sensorium, altered, 27
Serotonin selective reuptake inhibitors
   as preventive therapy, 106
Sexual activity, 156
Silberstein's classification, *111*
Single photon emission computed
   tomography (SPECT), 146
Sinus infection, 25
Sinusitis, emergency evaluation, 38
Sixth nerve palsy, 37, 43
Skew deviations, 73
Sleep alteration, 101, 143
Sleep pattern, 129–130
Sleeping difficulties, 9, 22
Source of pain, 48
Spacial distortions, 75
Sporting activity, 156
Sports injury, 175–176
Stiff neck, 27
   with fever, 38
Stress, 78, 101, 121
Stress management, 102, 133
Stressful environment, *23*

Stroke-like episodes, 160
Subarachnoid hemorrhage, 27, 170
Subarachnoid leak, 43
Substance abuse, 178
Substance-induced, emergency evaluation,
    39–40, 178
Substance P, 48–50
Sudden "thunderclap" headache, 27, 170
Sumatriptan
    dosage, acute, *91*, 98
    efficacy of, 89–91
    nasal spray, 91–92, 98
    recurrence rate, 90–91
    side effects, 90
    test dosages, 89–90
SUNCT, 52
Sweating, *82*
Symptoms
    associated, *23*
    localized, *22*
    progressive, 24
    spinal, 37
    warning, *22*
Syncope, *72*
Syndromes, 153–162
Syringomyelia, 37

Tachycardia, 37
Telescoping, 8
Temporal pattern, *21*
Temporomandibular joint disorder, 154–155
    jaw clicking, 154
Tension-type headache, 81, 117, 146
    episodic, *81*
    physiology, 121
Thalamus, 51–52
Thirst, 63
Thrombosis, 41
Tinnitus, 43, *72*
Tolosa-Hunt syndrome, 73
Transformed migraine, 14–15, 117, 118–119
Trauma, emergency evaluation, 40
Trazodone, 110
Treatment
    chronic daily headache, 121–123
        behavioral, 123
    nonpharmacologic, 126–141
    pharmacologic, 87–115, 139
        acute strategies, 88–98
        communication, 87, *111*
        re-evaluation, 87
    post-traumatic, 147–149
    psychologic, 126–141
        lifestyle modifications, 129–133
        reassurance, 126–127, 133–134, 139

Tricyclic antidepressants, 105, 148
    dosage, preventive, *104*
Trigeminal ganglion, 48–50
Trigeminal nucleus caudalis, 50
Trigeminal pain, modulation of, 52–53
Trigeminocervical complex, 50–51
Trigeminovascular anatomy, 48–49
Trigeminovascular physiology, 49–52
Triggers, *102*
    food, 101, 132
    identifying, 99–100
Triptans, 89–92, 148
    contraindications to, *96*
    mild to moderate migraine, 88–89
    moderate to severe migraine, *90*
    tablet limits, 88
Types of headache, *21*
    identifying, 20–32
    more than one, 21

Unilaterality, 3

Vahlquist criteria, 3–5, 61
Valproate sodium, 104
Vascular disorders
    emergency evaluation, 41–43
    frequency, 41
Vascular event, imaging for, 29
Vasculitis, 41
Venous obstruction, imaging for, 29
Venous sinus thrombosis, 42
Vertebro-basilar migraine, 71
Vertigo, 66, 71–73, 76, 143, 144
    abrupt appearance of, 66, 72
Visual difficulty, *23*, 27, 41, 43, 65–66, 71, *72*,
    75–76
Vomiting, 22 , 36–37, 60–64, *72*, 77, 79, 155,
    156
    cyclic, 78–79
    to dehydration, 78
    episodic, 78, 160
    pernicious, 78
    sudden, 72
    vigorous, 77–78

Warmth, *22*
Weakness, *23*, 41, 69, *72*
Withdrawal, 63–64
Worsening, *22*

Zolmitriptan
    dosage, acute, *91*, 92
    efficacy, 92, 98
Zomig
    dosage, acute, *91*, *92*